I Have WHAT???

MULTIPLE MYELOMA?!!
WALDENSTROM'S?!!
MACROGLOBULINEMIA?!!
AMYLOIDOSIS?!!
MGUS?!!

(Monoclonal Gammopathy of Undetermined Significance)

Written by Those Who Know!!!

By Debra Berenson

With an Introduction by Renowned Expert

Dr. James R. Berenson

ISBN-13: 978-0-9962359-2-1

DEDICATION

My beloved father, Wilford Arnovitz (MGUS), cousin Dr. Stanley Katz (multiple myeloma), and to all the patients and families who live with multiple myeloma, Waldenstrom's macroglobulinemia, amyloidosis and MGUS and to the doctors, scientists, nurses, and other healthcare professionals who help to make patients' lives better and continue to search for a cure.

All proceeds from the sale of this book will go to the Institute for Myeloma & Bone Cancer Research (IMBCR). The Institute is a 501(c)3 organization and your contribution is fully tax-deductible to the extent permitted by law.

Institute for Myeloma
& Bone Cancer Research

9201 West Sunset Boulevard, Suite 300

West Hollywood, CA 90069

310-623-1210   F 310-623-1120

contactus@imbcr.org

www.imbcr.org Tax ID # 46-0475333

ACKNOWLEDGEMENTS

My sincerest thank you to all of the patients and caregivers for sharing their most intimate thoughts regarding their experiences with multiple myeloma, Waldenstrom's macroglobulinemia, amyloidosis, and MGUS, and for their contributions to this book. We know that your input, and that of the doctors and other healthcare professionals, will be very helpful to everyone reading it!

Also, a special thanks to: Jenna Riehl, Executive Assistant to Dr. James Berenson; Tommy Garceau, Former Executive Assistant to Dr. James Berenson; Geoffrey Gee, Executive Director of the Institute for Myeloma & Bone Cancer Research; Tony Garzio, Chairman of the IMBCR Advisory Board; Paula DeYoung; Emilie Jackson; Susan Kolb; Dale Herd; Jody Furie; Rebecca Freidman; my mother, Barbara Arnovitz; my brother, David Arnovitz; our daughters Ariana Berenson and Shira Berenson Feinstein; our son-in-law, Dr. Aaron Feinstein; and, of course, to my husband, Dr. Jim Berenson, and to all of the other doctors, nurses, and healthcare professionals who contributed to this book and work tirelessly to treat patients with these diseases.

TABLE OF CONTENTS

FOREWORD

It is so gratifying to know that the first edition of the book has helped so many people! Many thanks to the people that have bought copies and have supported the cancer research being conducted in the IMBCR's laboratory with the proceeds from the sales of the book. Thank you to the people who have taken their time to write their appreciation in the many handwritten notes, emails, and Facebook posts I have received. It makes the seven years it took for me to go from "idea to book" a very worthwhile endeavor. I'm so happy that so many of you have found it a helpful resource for yourselves, your family, your caregivers, and/or your friends. I've enjoyed being interviewed about it, interviewing patients who provided stories in the book, and supplying copies to support groups and pharmaceutical companies—anything to help people realize that they can lead a "normal" life with these diseases and to help alleviate some of the anxiety that comes with getting one of these diagnoses.

The second edition will contain a few professionals that I know will only add to the book: Robert Dolgoff, MD Psychiatrist; Mary Donkersloot, RD Nutritionist; and Xiuling Ma, PhD OMD Acupuncturist. Also, included you'll find a few new chapters: Aliza G., Lawyer—In Memory of her Father; David K., Commercial Developer; Dale H., Screenwriter; Jay C., Basketball player; Steve B.,

Professor of Economics; and Phyllis G., Retired Teacher and Paralegal.

My husband, Dr. Jim Berenson, has specialized in treating patients with immune-based cancers, including multiple myeloma, Waldenstrom's macroglobulinemia, amyloidosis, and MGUS for more than 40 years. Jim and I have developed close relationships with many of his patients and some of our closest friends are the doctors who specialize in treating complications resulting from these cancers.

Because my father had MGUS and many other relatives and friends throughout the years have struggled with these diseases, I feel connected to the emotional path that Jim's patients are traveling. My hope is that this book will make the journey with your particular disease easier. Jim's close cousin, Stanley Katz, who was a very well-known and respected orthopedic surgeon in Los Angeles, was diagnosed with multiple myeloma in 1985. Ironically, he was a doctor who treated patients with bone problems, and he himself was stricken with a bone disease. Unfortunately, Stanley only lived two years following his diagnosis of myeloma, but that was back in 1985. Our cousin's struggle with myeloma propelled my husband to start working in this area more than 40 years ago. Today, Jim's patients are living so much longer—often 10, 15, and 25 years after being diagnosed! Both my husband and I are passionate about not only finding new and better treatments, but also finding a cure for these cancers that are currently incurable. Most importantly, Jim and the clinical staff in his practice focus on prolonging the lives of patients while at the same time improving their quality of life.

This book will shed light on these diseases using the perspectives of patients, their family members, and healthcare professionals. It will also serve as an easy-to-understand "medical book" for the newly diagnosed patient, as well as for their families and friends.

The first section contains accounts from patients who have been dealing with these disorders for some time. Originally, I hoped that the patients that shared their "war stories" would find writing down their experience cathartic and also that the newly diagnosed patient would find these patients' words of wisdom helpful. But, in reading the final product, I found a very hopeful and inspiring book filled with incredible strength and a strong will to live.

In the second part of the book, the doctors who treat problems associated with these disorders address how patients can manage complications from their particular disease and minimize side effects from their treatments. My hope is that the reader will benefit from having both of these perspectives and feel more confident in dealing with their own illness or that of a family member or friend who has one of these conditions. Most importantly, these accounts show that patients can have long and fulfilling lives after being diagnosed with multiple myeloma, Waldenstrom's macroglobulinemia, amyloidosis, or MGUS.

In 2004, my husband began caring for patients with these conditions in his own clinic, James R. Berenson, MD, Inc. in Los Angeles after spending two decades at the UCLA School of Medicine as a Professor in the Department of Medicine. He also founded the non profit Institute for Myeloma & Bone Cancer Research (IMBCR) in an adjacent facility. The Institute contains a basic research laboratory, which focuses on finding better ways to treat and follow patients with these forms of cancer. Jim and his hard-working team of scientists have discovered many new treatments for patients who now live longer and with better quality of life because of this work. He and his team strive to ultimately cure these diseases. Jim also formed a clinical trials organization, Oncotherapeutics, that performs studies to evaluate new treatments for his and other patients with these diseases around the world. This is the only model of its kind—a non-profit research institute, a medical practice, and a trials group focused on improving the lives of patients with these conditions, all under the same roof.

In the United States, more than 30,000 people are diagnosed each year with multiple myeloma and more than 150,000 Americans are living with this disease. New cases of Waldenstrom's macroglobulinemia (WM) occur in 3,000 Americans annually and more than 20,000 are living with this cancer. Amyloidosis occurs about as frequently as WM, but only about 10,000 Americans have it. MGUS is clearly very common and occurs in more than 3% of those over 50, 5% of those over 70, and nearly 10% of the population over

80 years of age. These patients are at higher risk to develop myeloma, WM, amyloidosis, and lymphoma.

I hope you find this book helpful and comforting and find that a full life is possible even with a diagnosis of these diseases. The patients and caregivers who shared their stories are very candid about what they have experienced. To keep their identities anonymous, only the initial of their last name appears.

If you find the book inspiring and Dr. Berenson's and his colleagues' philosophy and information on treating patients helpful, please consider donating to help further advance the research on these diseases at:

IMBCR.ORG -- "DONATE NOW"
Jenna Riehl -- jriehl@imbcr.org | 310-623-1214

IMBCR
9201 Sunset Boulevard, Suite 300
West Hollywood, California 90069

Thank you!

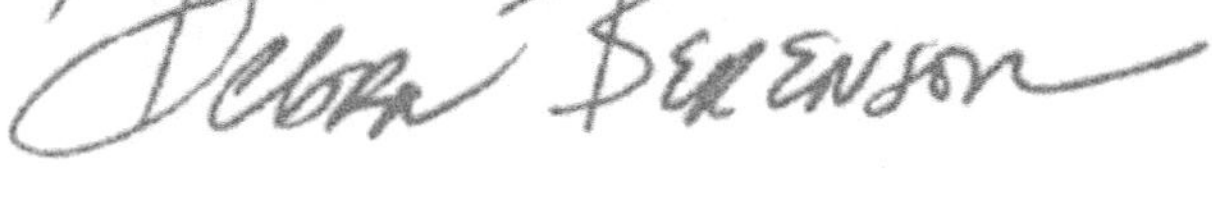

INTRODUCTION

By James R. Berenson, MD

Recently, new treatments that combat plasma cell disorders (i.e., multiple myeloma, its precursor monoclonal gammopathy of undetermined significance (MGUS), primary amyloidosis, and Waldenstrom's macroglobulinemia) have dramatically improved not only the survival but the quality of life of patients with these diseases. As a doctor and researcher dedicated to the care and improvement of the lives of these patients for more than three decades, it has been most heartening to be a part of these advances on both the basic research and clinical side of things.

At 12 years old, I was exposed to these diseases when I lost my father to cancer. I began my cancer research career working on immune therapies for leukemia during medical school, when I worked at the University of Washington under the guidance of Drs. Alexander Fefer and Donnall Thomas, the latter who went on to be awarded the Nobel Prize for his pioneering studies in bone marrow transplantation.

My specific interest in multiple myeloma stemmed from research during my fellowship in hematology and oncology at UCLA; at that time, I was studying the genes that produce antibodies from plasma cells, the types of cells that are the malignant culprits in multiple myeloma. Back then, not much work was being done on these disorders, especially basic science research, and the little that was being done had very limited relevance to patients. The only treatment options were chemotherapy and steroids, which resulted in much suffering during a lifespan that was usually measured in months.

Shortly after completing my fellowship and during my early years on faculty at UCLA, my wife Debra developed hand problems from her pregnancy with our older daughter Shira. My cousin Stanley Katz was a prominent Los Angeles-based orthopedic surgeon who cared for her with much kindness and expertise. While he was taking care of Debra, Stanley hugged his teenage son in the swimming pool and developed multiple rib fractures. Ironically, my cousin the bone doctor was soon found to have developed these problems from multiple myeloma, a cancer of the bone marrow. Stanley's treatments were limited to chemotherapy and steroids, and his courageous battle with myeloma was fraught with much suffering. He lost his fight after less than two years, which was about the average survival in the 1980s.

Because of my previous research work on immune therapy and studies of antibodies and plasma cells, I decided to dedicate myself to a career of finding ways to better understand and treat myeloma and related diseases. I wanted to help other patients be able to enjoy lives that would not be limited in length and quality by its devastating effects.

In the 1980s, myeloma was treated with chemotherapy drugs that were also used for a wide variety of unrelated cancers. Little emphasis was placed on trying to understand the biology in a way that would lead to better and more specific therapies for patients. Laboratory research had little connection with what went on in the clinic, and very little progress occurred to improve the length or quality of lives of myeloma patients.

In the 1990s, advances in molecular biology began to further our understanding of the specific genetic changes that occurred in myeloma cells. New treatment approaches were being developed using high dose chemotherapy followed by autologous transplantation; this resulted in deeper remissions and less myeloma remaining in the patient in comparison to conventional lower doses of chemotherapy. Some patients experienced lives that were myeloma free for long periods of time; however, for most, the experience was still one fraught with constant pain, with reductions in tumor burden that had, in fact, little impact on prolonging their lives.

It was also at this time that advances in supportive care began to be manifest in new treatments. They markedly improved the quality of lives of patients. The use of intravenous bisphosphonates administered on a monthly basis, first Aredia and more recently Zometa, led to a notable reduction in bone related problems, with fewer fractures and less bone pain, and a reduced need for pain medications, surgery, and radiation therapy. At the same time, drugs to stimulate red blood cell production such as Procrit and Aranesp were being shown to reduce the need for blood transfusions due to anemia or low red blood cell counts. Similarly, drugs to boost white blood cell counts such at first Neupogen followed by Neulasta reduced the risk of infection when blood counts were brought down to dangerously low levels from the effects of chemotherapy. But despite these advances and the panoply of new supportive care agents, no true anti-myeloma drugs were available.

At the end of the 1990s, it was serendipity that led to the first major advance in the treatment of the disease. A persistent New York lawyer and wife of a myeloma patient had heard about Dr. Judah Folkman's work at Harvard Medical School showing that it was possible to treat cancer with drugs that would block blood vessel formation in tumors. She was told that thalidomide, the drug that caused severe birth defects in babies whose mothers took it during pregnancy in the 1940s and 1950s, was capable of blocking blood vessel formation and became available for use because it was FDA-approved for treating another disease, leprosy. Although her husband, a patient at the University of Arkansas, did not respond, a second patient who was treated there showed a dramatic improvement in his myeloma after being treated with this drug. This rapidly led to an avalanche of studies demonstrating the effectiveness of thalidomide for patients who had failed to respond to other therapies. Finally, there was a drug that was effective for myeloma beyond the steroids and chemotherapy agents. However, like all drugs, this one came with a laundry list of side effects. Patients frequently experienced peripheral neuropathy which resulted in numbness, tingling, and sometimes pain in the hands and feet, and often somnolence (sleepiness).

As we entered the new millennium, there was a tremendous surge in myeloma research, with attempts to come up with drugs similar to thalidomide without these side effects, as well as develop new classes of drugs that would help myeloma patients. Velcade, a drug known as a proteasome inhibitor, initially developed for lupus and related auto immune disorders, was tried for patients with a variety of different cancers. It was found especially effective for treating myeloma patients, which led to clinical trials demonstrating its activity as a single agent and its subsequent initial approval for use in myeloma patients who had failed other treatments.

Next, attempts were made to combine these newer agents together and with older chemotherapy drugs and steroids in order to improve anti-myeloma properties without, most importantly, increasing their side effects. Our laboratory research and the work of others indicated lower doses of these agents could, in fact, be used effectively and safely when these drugs were combined together. This led to a series of clinical trials consistently showing the same results. Side effects varied among the different types of drugs, but the lower doses meant a reduction in side effects while still allowing patients to experience lives with better quality.

During this time, analogs, or similar drugs, to thalidomide and Velcade were also being developed with early promising results. Revlimid, an analog of thalidomide, showed better results with steroids than steroids alone and was also FDA approved in that combination to treat myeloma patients for whom other treatments had failed. These advances were reflected for the first time in my career with significant improvements in the survival of our patients, who were now beginning to expect to live in many cases for decades instead of a few years. These newer drugs eventually were studied in newly diagnosed myeloma patients, and the results of those trials led to the approval of these drugs for those patients as well.

Over the past few years, we have learned something new about these agents that was not part of our thinking in the early days of chemotherapy and steroids to treat myeloma: failure of one drug in combination does not mean that the same drug will not work in another treatment regimen. Even drugs that are very similar to one another can be substituted for one another with excellent anti-MM effects; for example, the newer proteasome inhibitor Kyprolis is often effective for treating patients who have failed Velcade. Similar findings are also observed with the newest analog of thalidomide, Pomalyst, showing that patients failing thalidomide or Revlimid often respond to this newer version. These findings have dramatically increased the treatment options for patients, which has resulted in an ever-increasing smorgasbord of therapeutic choices that are available for our patients today. This not only means that patients failing to respond to a particular treatment can also try a myriad of different regimens. It also indicates that if they perhaps respond to but do not tolerate a particular drug or combination, they can know there is something else out there on the horizon to try.

Advances in the laboratory are furthering our understanding of the biology of these diseases and allowing us to predict outcomes for our patients based on their specific genetic makeup. But this has not yet been translated into risk-adapted therapies, or treatments that can be given to a patient based solely on these genetic characteristics. Importantly, for the first time, we are moving into the era of trying to target the myeloma cell itself without allowing the therapy to be active anywhere else in the body. Monoclonal antibodies that target the myeloma cell and at the same time boost the immune system are for the first time showing effectiveness for treating myeloma patients. The goal of this treatment approach is to accomplish what I could only imagine when my wife's acting producer and director Geo Hartley, a founding board member at the Institute for Myeloma & Bone Cancer Research, said to her many years ago: "It's not about more; it's about being more specific." It's that specificity that will lead us to what we all hope for our patients—treatment that gets rid of myeloma once and for all without having any impact on the rest of the body, so that patients can know they will experience full lives untouched by the effects of myeloma.

THE PATIENTS

I Have WHAT???

By Aliza G. -- MULTIPLE MYELOMA?!!
In loving memory of her father, David K.

Age: 80's

Commercial Developer

My father was always afraid of serious illness. Hospitals and very sick people made him uncomfortable and scared. I always hoped that when his time came to die, he would go quickly. But that did not happen: he got Multiple Myeloma and did what he hated and feared for many years—suffering with pain and experiencing a diminishing quality of life.

Dad shrunk from 5'9½" to under 5'6" quickly, and no one picked up on why. His diaphragm broke. He had mesh Gore-Tex surgically inserted between his stomach and his chest because they were collapsing on each other. Still no why. Then the phone rang one day while I was on another continent in a hotel on vacation. It was Dad saying that he had cancer and that I could tell no one but close family.

My father would not let us help him decide on his care. After interviewing a number of doctors, he chose a general oncologist rather than a specialist in Multiple Myeloma. Why? He did not tell me who he was seeing or what his decision process was. He was in increasing pain with compression fractures in his vertebrae. He still went to work and kept his cancer a secret. He was always private and cared about his image. I think that he did not want to seem weak or scare other people. He did not want people feeling sorry for him or treating him as less than whole.

After several years, my dad's cancer got worse and he realized that he needed more expert and specialized care. This is when he became a patient of Dr. Jim Berenson. The funny thing was that I knew Jim because our kids were friends and we were friends. But I never knew all the time what kind of cancer he worked on.

Jim did a great job for my dad. He was caring and patient. Jim gave him his cell phone number and was there for us 24/7. He was on the leading edge of Myeloma care and knew all the options and latest advances. He exercised great judgment in helping my dad decide on what to do.

My dad eventually went on trials of experimental drugs. Some helped. Some made him feel terrible.

During one of his stays in the hospital my Dad contracted MRSA (methicillin resistant staph infection). It really took the air and the hope out of him. It was hard to watch. He was in intensive care for several weeks and some doubted he would survive, but he recovered. Still, he was in and out of the hospital regularly after that event. He had a wonderful full-time nurse at home, but he experienced little joy out of life. He started giving up the fight. He wondered whether all the additional pills, trips to the doctors, and drips were worth it. His grandchildren were his greatest joy and the reason he got up every morning.

I miss my father and think of him every day, though he died 12 years ago. I wonder what he would think of his kids and grandkids if he could see them today. I think that he would be pleased and proud.

I Have WHAT???

By Alma B. -- MULTIPLE MYELOMA?!!

Age: 70s

Educator and Photographer

I know you all must have experiences, hopes, and dreams to share.

I'm really glad for the opportunity to describe my experience of what it is like to be a multiple myeloma patient and how I've benefited by participating in clinical trials under the direction of my doctor and friend—Dr. Berenson.

One Saturday morning, in the summer of 1996, my husband Aaron and I decided to hike up Signal Hill. It's a steep rise overlooking the port of Long Beach, CA. Puff! Puff! "This is hard! I must get myself in condition. This won't do!"

One afternoon, several weeks later, I was busy with errands and was so hot and tired. I just wanted to go home, have a glass of orange juice, and relax in my recliner.

Wow! It was good to be home and be in that chair, but, "What's this? I'm having trouble breathing and talking. I feel terrible! What's happening to me?"

Fortunately, my husband was sitting near me and noticed my distress. He dialed 911 and soon I was at the local hospital. I was admitted to the ICU and stayed there for two days with a lot of testing. When I became stable, I was moved to another large hospital and settled into an attractive room.

My local doctor came in and gave me the news that I had multiple myeloma. Aaron was with me. The doctor thought I'd burst into tears, but there were too many questions, such as: What is it? And how could it be treated?

At home, the unwelcome turn of events sunk in. Of course, we were very sad and upset that our lives would now be changed forever. We cried and held each other.

Then, we began reading everything we could to learn about multiple myeloma. When I became too depressed, I quit reading, but Aaron persisted and also began checking around for the best doctor. And was I ever lucky—he found Dr. Berenson!

In mid-September, we went to meet with Dr. Berenson. He and his staff very carefully explained treatment choices, related protocols, potential benefits and risks to me. I agreed to a stem cell transplant and things happened fast. The first of three rounds of VAD chemotherapy started. Plans were to have a stem cell transplant as part of a clinical trial in early January.

The trial would study variations in the stem cell transplant procedures. Why enter into such a trial? For me, the reasons were compelling. My cancer was already Stage 3—the most severe stage of myeloma, so aggressive that intervention with a transplant seemed right.

From a larger perspective my undergoing a stem cell transplant procedure at all was because earlier researchers and patients had made the decision to take part in clinical trials. It was now my turn.

I entered my first clinical trial with much hope. My primary pre-transplant treatment was called VAD—three letters which stand for three very strong medications. The D component of VAD was dexamethasone, dex for short. Dex is a steroid. It really energized me, sometimes at the wrong time. It gave us laughs as I zipped around the house doing neglected chores.

One job was cleaning the exterior of the oven—not the interior which could involve chemicals dangerous to me. Well, I scrubbed and scrubbed. When I finished, I saw that I had completely rubbed off the numbers on the oven dial. Gee!

Another day I went into action thoroughly cleaning, drying, and rehanging all 40 pieces of the small glass chandelier above our dining room table. It had to be done, so it was!

Many evenings I stayed up late because I was so wired that it was hard to fall asleep. Luckily, I wasn't required to take the 10 dex pills every day in the cycle. Have you known anyone on dex? If so, then you could tell stories, too.

During this time, I had several visits with Dr. Berenson monitoring how I was doing. A home health care nurse checked me, too. Everything seemed to be going well. I only became anxious about the transplant about a week before entering the hospital.

The day—January 1, 1999—came. Aaron drove me to the hospital. I settled into my tenth-floor room with lots of things to do—books to read, cards to send out, and tape recordings to listen to. By the second day I felt trapped in that room and depressed to know I couldn't get out of there, but in a few days, after the transplant, that didn't even matter. I was too tired to do much of anything. I slept a lot. My throat was very sore.

That January brought rain almost daily. As I recovered from the procedure, I looked out of my hospital window and watched the rain pouring down. Aaron stayed with me as much as he could and helped me keep my spirit up. The 20 days passed and I was happy to return home.

My myeloma numbers were greatly reduced. I regained strength slowly, but in June I was well enough to visit my family in Kentucky and Ohio. One day I went with my sister-in-law to a water aerobics class. The other students looked me over. I had lost all of my hair in treatment, but by now I had a little bit of hair all over my scalp. One woman looked at me and asked, "Is that a California style?" I explained. (It was the time of the *G.I. Jane* movie, so short, short hair wasn't *completely* out of style.) By September, I felt much stronger. Aaron and I went hiking in Glacier National Park. I loved that trip.

Of course, I was grateful for the return to normalcy. I benefited so much from that clinical trial. For two years, I didn't need anything else to sustain the good results. For three years after that I only took steroids, before another treatment was necessary.

From that clinical trial, I really benefited in three important ways. First, I was under the watchful care of some of the world's finest physicians and researchers. Second, I was knocking down the myeloma. Third, it brought me several years of life while other treatments were being developed. When I was first diagnosed in the mid-nineties, there weren't many options, but within a few years, whole new treatments had been researched and were in use.

In November 2002, I required another kind of treatment to bring down my rising myeloma numbers. Dr. Berenson, Aaron, and I discussed the choices. I signed the consent papers for the clinical trial using the drugs Velcade and melphalan. With this new chemotherapy,

I felt some nausea. My muscles, especially my chest muscles, seemed to get pulled easily, but overall I found the treatment quite tolerable. It was effective for about a year. That clinical trial certainly benefited me, giving me another year of good-quality life.

Next, I signed on for a clinical trial called MAC, which stands for melphalan, arsenic trioxide, and vitamin C. Side effects such as headaches, rashes, and some infections were all manageable. The MAC combination helped me for about nine months.

Now I could tell you about the other clinical trials I was part of, but you wouldn't want to hear all of that. I will tell you their treatment names:

- SGN-40 (an antibody trial)
- Doxil, dexamethasone, arsenic trioxide, and vitamin C
- Velcade and samarium—a radioactive substance
- Organic arsenic—different from the other arsenic
- arsenic and Velcade

Please know that each of these was a clinical trial. Some worked, others didn't, but all were tolerable and bought time. I'm certain they all added to the body of knowledge on myeloma.

Yes, being on some clinical trials gave me unpleasant experiences—rashes, headaches, pulled muscles, mouth thrush, urinary tract infections and, of course, the bone marrow biopsies. These were no fun at all, but were dealt with, did end, and life was still a joy.

It has been interesting to have the opportunity to talk with and get to know other patients. I've made several good friends at the clinic. We encourage each other. Aaron, my family, and friends have given me much love and support. They all have played a big part in my well-being and cheer me on.

I thank Dr. Berenson and the other fine researchers who use their knowledge in creative ways to venture into the unknown and perhaps come up with a new solution.

I was on many clinical trials. Each trial has directly or indirectly led to improved treatment, survival and quality of life. I hope these trials will bring us closer to cures in the future. That is why funding is so important.

I hope that in reading this in some way you've been motivated to help others. Maybe you have a relative or friend who is a blood disease patient. Perhaps you are a patient.

Whatever the case, I thank each of you for all of your work which has helped to make life-saving treatments a reality. I appreciate everyone's great effort to make good things happen for me and other patients.

I Have WHAT???

By Alvin D. -- MULTIPLE MYELOMA?!!

Age: 80s

Retired Vice President of a department store

Every morning, now, when I look in the mirror, I say, "Wow, you are a very lucky guy!" You might ask, "Why—why does he say this? Sounds pretty strange."

Let me tell you a story. Eighteen years ago, my internist took a chest x-ray. Big deal, we all have annual chest x-rays.

This was different. The doctor said, "You have a lump on your rib. We must do a needle biopsy." They did the needle biopsy and found nothing.

My doctor used some ugly words and then said, "Do the biopsy again!" I said, "No!" My doctor and my wife insisted. I lost the argument, but won my life due to the early discovery of my cancer. They told me the second biopsy showed a form of multiple myeloma.

What do you do after you are told you have a diagnosis of cancer? Well, you call your college friends, fraternity brothers, and all the doctors that you know to find the top specialists in the country at Mayo Clinic, Harvard, Arkansas, MD Anderson, etc.

As a result of my friends' connections, a chief oncologist at the University of Washington called me back. I will now quote him: "You idiot. You don't have to go all over the country. The most brilliant doctor in the United States in the area of multiple myeloma is Dr. James Berenson, right there in LA."

Others confirmed what he had said. My doctor friend at UCLA got an appointment for me in two days.

That is when the miracle began. In July of 1994 at 64 years of age, I had my first treatment for multiple myeloma: eight weeks of radiation, 40 times in total, plus an infusion of Aredia (a bone strengthener) every 28 days. Now I receive an even more powerful bone strengthener called Zometa every month.

The cancer next reappeared on my chest bone. They cut out this lesion, and I was given seven weeks of radiation, 35 times in total.

Things always come in threes. The cancer then reappeared in my collar bone. This time, it was treated with surgery and four weeks of radiation, 20 times in total.

All during this time, Dr. Berenson was so positive that I would be okay. I am now approaching 82 years of age. Dr. Berenson made my life a positive experience.

That is not the end of my story. Dr. James Berenson introduced me to Dr. Jacob Zighelboim who gave me the power to meditate, visualize, and psychologically handle my cancer.

Then, just to keep things exciting in my life, I developed prostate cancer. Again, Dr. Berenson helped, this time by giving me the names of the outstanding professionals in this field. My prostate cancer is now in remission.

I can't stop now. I had a heart attack on the way to one of my Zometa treatments. Dr. Berenson took an electrocardiogram and sent me to a heart specialist. They inserted a stent.

Wait a minute, I can't stop now. Dr. Berenson, during a routine exam, noticed an irregular heartbeat. He sent me to another outstanding cardiologist who specialized in putting in pacemakers. After months of testing, the cardiologist installed a pacemaker.

If you are old enough to remember a movie called *Miracle on 34th Street*, you will see that my miracle is on Sunset Boulevard in Dr. Berenson's office. How lucky can you get?! First, in finding a warm, caring, and highly qualified Dr. James Berenson to treat my cancer, and then he gives you 18 years of life to see your son get married and have a son and a daughter (my 5-year-old grandson and his 19-month-old sister).

Thank you, Dr. Berenson, for giving me the time to experience all the joys of my life.

P.S. My wife Barbara insisted that I follow Dr. Berenson's instructions to the letter. They both made it possible for me to last 18 years, and I am still going strong.

So there you have it: "the story of a very lucky guy."

I Have WHAT???

By Anastasia M. B. -- MULTIPLE MYELOMA?!!

In loving memory of her father, Rev. Fr. E. V. M., Ph.D.

Age: 70s

Greek Orthodox Priest

I will never forget the day that I first heard the words multiple myeloma. It was a crisp and bright day in Southern California. It was the first week of January 1996. I was 4 months pregnant and working in my office waiting for a phone call from my parents. My father had gone in for his yearly physical a few weeks earlier and his doctor had found an irregularity in his blood work. In his characteristic way, my dad told me that there was a slight abnormality. Although more tests were being ordered, he reassured me it wasn't a problem and not to worry. Of course, I did nothing but worry. On this particular day, my parents were meeting with my father's doctor to learn the outcome of the tests. The phone rang and I rushed to answer it. My mother was crying and told me that my dad had multiple myeloma and that the doctor was immediately sending them to an oncologist for a bone marrow biopsy and more tests. She told me that there was no cure. I asked to speak to my dad. Again, my dad, the eternal optimist, told me that everything would be fine and not to worry. I hung up the phone. My first thought was that my child might never have the opportunity to know my remarkable father, or experience the unconditional love that my father had given me, and then I started crying.

Of course, I immediately tried to find out everything that I could about this form of cancer that I had never heard of before. I told my dad that he had to go to a doctor who specialized in the disease as, at that time, it was relatively uncommon. My parents received a recommendation and met with an oncologist who treated multiple myeloma and other cancers. She told my parents that multiple myeloma was a type of cancer for which there wasn't a cure. She recommended that my dad start his treatment with a stem cell transplant and told him that his life expectancy with multiple myeloma was four to five years, and that he could die from the transplant itself. My dad was very quiet after this meeting as he tried to process what he had just been told. He liked the doctor but wasn't comfortable with the treatment that she proposed. We later talked about how there were huge differences in the way doctors approached the treatment of multiple myeloma, and that he had to make sure that he selected a physician who would treat his cancer while at the same time preserved his quality of life. While my parents were sitting in the oncologist's office waiting for my father's appointment, my sister-in-law saw a brochure on the wall about multiple myeloma. On the back cover of the brochure was the name of the man who, for the next 11 years, would try different combinations of treatments to prolong and preserve the quality of my dad's life, a man who would become my dad's trusted physician and friend, Dr. James Berenson.

My dad's first meeting with Dr. Berenson was very different from the meeting with the other oncologist. Dr. Berenson did not speak of life expectancies or drastic treatments. He told my dad that while there is no cure for multiple myeloma, it is highly treatable and that he had many patients who lived full lives for many years. Dr. Berenson repeated the bone marrow biopsy, took X-rays, and ran blood tests. He told my dad that given the facts that he had no symptoms, his bones did not yet have any lesions, and his myeloma protein marker in the blood, IgG, was at a relatively low level, he wasn't even going to call it active multiple myeloma, and he recommended that he simply monitor his condition every few months by simply performing blood and urine tests. If it did progress, Dr. Berenson assured him that there were many drugs available to comfortably treat the disease and that he and others were constantly researching and discovering new drugs and combinations of drugs that could work for my dad. My dad was thrilled. For many months, he proudly told us that he did not even have multiple myeloma.

My dad and Dr. Berenson valiantly fought this disease. It started slowly, and my dad enjoyed many years with minimal treatment. Throughout his battle with multiple myeloma, he was able to continue to tirelessly serve his parish, travel to his homeland of

Greece with us, and become as indispensable to my daughter Emily's life as he was to mine. As his disease progressed, he saw Dr. Berenson more frequently. My mother and Emily accompanied him on most of those appointments and I would go whenever I could. We were all very anxious before each of my dad's appointments and either relieved or worried after, depending on whether the IgG levels and kidney blood tests, creatinine numbers, went up or down. My dad tried everything that Dr. Berenson offered him and participated in many clinical trials. Dr. Berenson always told him not to worry; if a particular combination of drugs didn't work, he would try something else. As the years passed, new drugs and therapies became available, and with Dr. Berenson always at the forefront of these new therapies, my dad was able to reap their benefits quickly.

In the fall of 2005, my dad's multiple myeloma started resisting the treatment. He was also experiencing the effects of living with multiple myeloma for so long. His bones had new lesions, and he had lost nearly six inches in height from compression fractures in his spine. He underwent his first of two kyphoplasty surgeries. My dad was in pain and was very concerned, but he remained optimistic and determined. Dr. Berenson encouraged him and kept trying new and different combinations to stop the myeloma. But in January 2006, my dad's body started its decline. He was hospitalized for high potassium and creatinine levels. My own family had moved away from Los Angeles and was now living in Seattle, Washington. We flew down to be with him.

I will never forget that night when Dr. Berenson walked into my dad's hospital room with a smile and told him, "Don't worry, Father, this combination didn't work, but I am developing another one. I think that I am going to call it BAMA." My dad smiled, looked at us, and told us, "See, you don't have to worry, Dr. Berenson will find the right drugs for me." Indeed, Dr. Berenson gave my dad much hope during those last months of his life and never stopped trying to find a way to halt the progression of his myeloma.

Over the course of the next few months, we traveled to Los Angeles every three weeks to be with my dad. We went to his appointments and sat with him in the treatment chairs while he received his infusions. We met his friends who sat in the neighboring chairs. They were John and Alma. My dad would go to lunch with John in the coffee shop downstairs from Dr. Berenson's office. They would talk about their treatments, but they would also talk about their fears and their hopes. Alma shared my dad's passion for photography. She kept a journal of her treatments and she and my dad would share their experiences with the disease. She and my dad took arsenic around the same time. It didn't work for my dad but it was working for Alma. She was such a kind and special person.

During the last months of my dad's life, his kidneys failed and he began dialysis treatments. He was also experiencing more pain in his spine and in his pelvis. For the first time in 11 years, Dr. Berenson told my dad that he should enjoy his family and think about retiring. My dad continued to serve his parish with the assistance of substitute priests. His immune system was compromised and he couldn't climb stairs easily, but he would still go to the hospital to visit sick parishioners. He went to every service at his church even if he could only sit in the altar. On August 15, 2006, my dad went to his last appointment with Dr. Berenson. He wanted to come to Seattle to be with us. Dr. Berenson advised him not to go. My dad needed an MRI and Dr. Berenson wanted to be able to take care of him, but my dad wanted to be with us and especially with his beloved Emily. My dad was adamant and left Dr. Berenson with no choice. Dr. Berenson called a colleague in Seattle and made all of the necessary arrangements to make sure that my dad had the best care during what would turn out to be the last weeks of his life.

My dad died at Virginia Mason Medical Center at 1:15 a.m. on September 22, 2006. My mother and I were by his side. Three days before he died, he insisted that I call two people on their cell phones. One was Dr. Berenson. He wanted to thank him. I held the phone for him as he told Dr. Berenson that he was the best physician and thanked him for keeping him alive for so long.

Although my dad ultimately lost his battle with multiple myeloma, the determination with which he lived his life, fought his disease, and faced his death serves as an example for all who had the privilege to know him or learn about him. His story is a story of hope, faith, and profound love. Perhaps the best way to describe how he felt about Dr. Berenson and multiple myeloma is to share his own words. Dr. and Mrs. Berenson attended the 41st Anniversary Celebration of my dad's ordination to the priesthood. At that celebration, my father said:

> *"I want to pay tribute and recognize the man who extended my life and my ministry, my beloved medical doctor James R. Berenson, a great researcher, a recognized authority all over the world on multiple myeloma, a physician with a human touch, and a determined healer."*

At that same celebration, my father reflected on his multiple myeloma diagnosis:

> *In the course of my ministry, eight years ago this month, I was diagnosed with multiple myeloma, a cancer of the bone marrow. It was a severe test of my strength and of everything I built for so many years. I was very aware of all of the potential risks that come with having multiple myeloma, particularly the risk to my life. However, I prayed and I thanked God for the challenge. I was immediately faced with ultimate questions. Nevertheless, as I overcame fear and strengthened myself, I found hope with help from my Presvytera Maria, Stacey and Bill and their families, and with the arrival of Emily in our lives, rays of a bright sunshine enlighten my life, and from an inner strength that was my faith, my entire ministry took a new turn. I would like to quote Victor E. Frankl from his famous book,* Man's Search for Meaning: *"The way in which a man accepts his fate and all the suffering it entails, the way in*

which he takes up his cross, gives him ample opportunity—even under the most difficult circumstances—to add a deeper meaning to his life."

. . .

One of the greatest contemporary poets of Greece, George Seferis, always captivated my mind with his powerful existential interpretation of man's destiny and his universal spirit. In one of his poems, Seferis writes:

'A little farther,
We will see the almond trees blossoming.
The marble gleaming in the sun.
The sea breaking into waves.
A little farther,
Let us rise a little higher.'

According to the vision of the poet, who masterfully captures the infinite strength of man to always rise like the mythical phoenix from the ashes, all our efforts, all our prayers, all our agonies, all our personal and family anxieties focused on one single goal, to try just a little more to see the human heart blossom, to become whiter than the marble of the poet and to gleam in the sun of mercy, to be filled with feeling, human feeling, becoming subtle, a waving sea, embracing our fellow men and by rising a little farther and higher to fulfill the fatherhood of God and the brotherhood of man.

This is the precious legacy that my father instilled in me during his time on this earth. My father's example has compelled me to do something more with my time. Therefore, as a fitting tribute to his memory, in February 2012, I joined the Board of The Institute for Myeloma and Bone Cancer Research and am devoting my energy to help Dr. Berenson in his noble efforts to find a cure for multiple myeloma.

I Have WHAT???

By Arnie N. -- MGUS?!!

Age: 70s

Plumbing Supply Salesman

First thing I should say is that Dr. Berenson treats all of his patients like family. Also, he has a great bedside manner and he actually loves all the people who come in to see him. He deals with patients with honesty and a great loving attitude. He also jokes with all of us. Now I can say that my experience with Dr. Berenson is in a loving nature and we kid with each other all the time. And if anybody needs an oncologist, with this doctor you have a great one—probably the best in California and then some. Going to Dr. Berenson was the best decision I have made.

I Have WHAT???

By Bernie B. -- MULTIPLE MYELOMA?!!

Age: 90s

Businessman

I tell everyone that I owe my life to Dr. Berenson. He didn't just save my life…he gave my life back to me. Because when this story begins, I wasn't really living. I was existing. I was killing time, and time was killing me.

Let's go back a while, and see if I can string together the unraveled threads of illness that eventually brought me to Dr. Berenson's office, weak and ailing. I had the will to live— hat has never been a problem with me, with a positive attitude and a toughness that won't quit, and surrounded by loving family and loyal friends—but I didn't have the wherewithal. Although it might be simplifying things a bit, it's no exaggeration to say, underneath the smart clothing my beautiful wife Judy buys for me, I was a mess. My internal organs probably looked like a battle zone. My test results probably read like bad news from the front.

For about 10 to 15 years before this story began, I had a blood disease called polycythemia. This is a slow-growing type of blood disorder in which your bone marrow makes too many red blood cells. These excess cells thicken your blood and cause complications, such as a risk of blood clots or bleeding. Just like so many diseases I had, it isn't very common.

I had not been feeling myself for a while when my primary doctor and friend, Dr. K., told me that I would need a valve replacement in my heart. I was bleeding internally. We tried to find a doctor who would do this in a minimally invasive way, through the groin. Hard to imagine that anything "through the groin" could be minimally invasive, but it was considered the safest and least painful option.

While looking for a doctor, and for a valve that could fit me, a tallish man after all, the internal bleeding was too dangerous and I underwent surgery to remove a small area of the colon. Cancer. It was always cancer. I have lost track of how many cancers I have. Maybe that's part of what kept my spirits up. I always felt there was no cancer tougher than me, so what's the point in keeping track. Just take it out!

Next on the agenda was the open-heart surgery in which I received the valve I needed for my heart. The operation was successful from the standpoint of living and dying. I was at Cedars-Sinai and not Hillside Cemetery, so there was *that* to be thankful for, I suppose. But I was in no condition to be philosophical.

I had already stopped being "me." My family tells me I was "out of it" night and day, just sleeping, lying or staring at the ceiling. I have no memory of it. These years were like my Dark Ages, a long nothingness that seemed to have no beginning or end. I was existing, but for what? Waiting for a miracle? Maybe my family was, but like I said, it was all I could do to smile and hope for the best.
It was blind hope, I might add, because nothing that was happening to me gave me any reason for optimism. Except, of course, my wife's smile and her touch as she held my hand and helped me get through each difficult day. I have always said "Yes, Dear" to almost any request she has made of me during our 43 years of marriage. But if I needed any reminder of how dear she really is, I got it, over and over; as she made sure I ate enough, slept enough, took the right pills, and stayed comfortable through this terrible time in my life.

All the love in the world though couldn't seem to make me better; my weight fell from 175 to 123 pounds— and I'm six feet tall! You can imagine what I looked like. No one knew what was wrong. I saw doctors, and doctors saw me, but it was like we were ships passing in the night.

Much later I found out I had contracted a staph infection from one of the doctors who had performed the heart valve surgery, who if you can believe it had a sore on his hand and did not take the proper measures to prevent contamination! I never seem to have gotten angry at this oversight. Maybe it's because I was too weak to feel much emotion at all. Maybe it's because I understand that in this world, nobody's perfect. Clearly he did not make this mistake purposefully. I'm sure if he could relive the day of my surgery to spare me the life-threatening infection that ensued, he would.

Months passed. It seemed years. I just floated along in a sort of non-life. I'm sure I had lucid moments. I'm sure I must have enjoyed visits from my family and friends and must have shared meaningful moments with them, but for the life of me, I can't remember. During that time, my life was all one big blur and all about blood. I needed many blood transfusions, but sometimes I still had too many red cells in my blood. I would need a phlebotomy to remove blood requiring frequent trips to the hospital, and then sometimes I would need a transfusion, over and over and over again.

Eventually, we were sent to UCLA where my hematologist diagnosed me with multiple myeloma. Of course this was our first "I have WHAT?" moment. It sounded more like melanoma. We were advised to have a bone marrow test. The office made an appointment for the next day, but when we arrived for the procedure, there was no record of it. More insult added to more injury, I guess.

We went back to the hematologist's office without having the test done and he just said, "Look, you have multiple myeloma, the thing is now to start treating it." It didn't quite feel right to me, or my inner medical circle. It wasn't exactly that I was receiving slipshod treatment, but my confidence was not encouraged by the attention—

or should I say, lack of attention—I was getting from my doctor at that time. How could a doctor be so nonchalant with a nearly 90-year-old man suffering from a number of cancers and diseases, with multiple myeloma at the top of my list? Still, not knowing what else to do but growing more discontented day by dark day, we made a plan for weekly appointments, and three visits a week which was, to start the following month.

Finally, I did have the bone marrow test and was then told conclusively that I had multiple myeloma. I still did not completely comprehend the implications of this. I knew that strides had been made lately and that patients were surviving much longer now than just a few years ago, but what was my course of action to be? My wife was proactive and took the steps that ultimately would lift me out of the dark well that I had been living in: She called her best friend Donna. Thank G-d for Donna. And her friend knew Dr. Berenson, and this friend, in fact, told me that he owed his own life to the man.

My family doctor actually knew very little about him. However, once we looked into Dr. B's resume, met with him a few times, and discovered his impressive background and accolades, it was pretty clear he was a grownup prodigy, a maverick who was not afraid to speak his mind on what he thought would be best for me. No matter that he was no longer a young man (except compared to me!), he had a wunderkind's attitude and penchant for miracles. Somehow I knew he was going to fix the broken-down jalopy I had become. Somehow he would find the parts, or make me work without them.

That is exactly what he did.

At first, Dr. Berenson was challenged trying to establish medicines for me that would control my myeloma. Prior to my diagnosis of multiple myeloma, I had been on a new drug for treating polycythemia called Jakafi but it had not really provided me much good. Dr. Berenson took me off the drug when I started treatment for my myeloma because the drugs used to fight the myeloma also make blood counts go down just like Jakafi. When my myeloma did not respond to the therapies, my wife suggested to Dr. Berenson that maybe we should try Jakafi, a kinase inhibitor typically used in the treatment of polycythemia and other diseases in which too much is made. He agreed to add this to my conventional treatment with Revlimid and steroids. I would be the first patient in Dr. Berenson's practice (and probably the first in the entire world) who was on this combination! Luckily enough, he could only get the Jakafi paid for because of my polycythemia for which the drug is often used. Who knew that having polycythemia *and* multiple myeloma would turn out to be two strokes of good luck?

The treatment worked. Boy, did it work and more importantly it continues to work today, several years later. I feel great now.

Now each week I get a blood test, during which my myeloma protein levels are checked as well as my blood counts, and Dr. Berenson adjusts my medicine. My blood thinner also gets adjusted by Dr. K with the results from the same tests. My wife says, triumphantly, "And together, they put Humpty Dumpty back together again." No King's horses. No King's men. Just a group of smart medical folks at the top of their game.

This new treatment was studied at the Institute for Myeloma & Bone Cancer Research which Dr. Berenson leads. It has been so effective in the research laboratory that a clinical trial is starting now to evaluate this treatment in many myeloma patients throughout the United States.

If you notice, the story of my decline and fall is much longer than the story of my return to the land of the living. I think it's always that way when we are faced with obstacles, even the seemingly insurmountable ones. Suffering can go on a long time, and then it's over quick, one way or another. Dr. Berenson has shown me that with my myeloma (and with yours, whoever you are, whether you've been diagnosed yet or not) it's not a death sentence! It's not a life sentence either. For me, it has been a reversal of the sentence entirely. I plan to live forever; if anyone can arrange it, Dr. Berenson can.

In the meantime, I owe him my life. It seems forever ago that I couldn't focus on the simplest task. It's no exaggeration to say I couldn't even add one plus one. And now I can do what I have loved to do all my life. Work on my business. Interact with colleagues. Exercise. Go out to lunch with friends and have dinner with my family. Take care of the charities that are so meaningful to me and my wife. Explore the future. Just recently I got dropped off at the Milken Institute's Global Conference and spent the days wandering around like a kid in a candy store.

Like a kid. Who has his whole life in front of him. Which I do, thanks to my loving family, caring doctors, and of course, Dr. Berenson.

I Have WHAT???

By Bennett K. -- WALDENSTROM'S?!! and AMYLOIDOSIS?!!

Age: 70s

Attorney

I fell off my bike. It was August 1991. I was merely pedaling slowly up a small hill in Mendocino, California, while on vacation with my wife. My legs just gave out on me. I was adjacent to a grassy part of the hill, so I just fell sideways and gently landed on the dirt.

Two days earlier, while driving up the coast from our home in Los Angeles, we stopped at a lighthouse. I wanted to dash up its steps to the top. I got to the top, but had stopped dashing long before reaching it, my legs having grown very tired.

A few weeks earlier I ran (slowly) in a 6K race. Although not a runner, I had been athletic for many years. I finished the race, but could barely stand up afterwards, exhausted beyond expectation.

Earlier in March of that same year, I had participated in a handball tournament, having played handball for decades. I did okay in the tournament, enjoying the sport as usual. But what was of interest was that my legs had become very tired during the singles competition. That had never been a problem before.

I thought nothing of these separate occurrences, attaching no significance to these apparently unrelated events.

At least not until August 30, 1991, when I received blood test results after a routine physical exam. My internist advised that he had bad news and good news. The bad news was that I had a blood cancer. The good news was that it was Waldenstrom's macroglobulinemia (WM), an indolent, slow-moving form of cancer that is in the bone marrow and lymph glands. So, I now knew the answer to the previously unthought-of questions regarding why my legs started giving out beginning in March: I had a type of cancer that was causing me to be anemic.

Everyone has a story of what preceded their finding out that they had cancer. One's story is most interesting, of course, to oneself, and may possibly be of minimal interest to anyone else. However, what is most interesting to me is to have discovered at age 53 that my body was possessed by some kind of a "creature" over which I had no influence. It was controlling the way I lived, felt, and functioned. I was scared and angry, but mostly scared, and felt distressingly vulnerable. I did not know how indolent the disease was going to be, but, hopefully, thought that if it was slow-moving enough, medical science would be able to catch up and overtake it.

That is what has happened, thanks to the next doctor who entered this story, described below. After we met, I was able to add to my existing feelings those of quiet resolution and optimism.

The "literature" at the time advised that one had an average of a five-year life expectancy from diagnosis. Of course, the "literature" has been rewritten as I progressed through my treatment, which has now gone on and off for 24 years.

My internist, a friendly acquaintance from college, referred me to Dr. James Berenson, who has become more than a friendly acquaintance over the years. Indeed, we have grown (much) older together. Jim has benefitted from being exposed to my sparkling personality. I have benefitted more so, however, not only from his, but because, as a result of his thoughtful and skilled care and caring, I am still around to write about my experiences with this disease.

When we first started together, I needed immediate treatment. He (we) settled on a course that was successful, allowing me to stop treatment after two years, not needing to resume any treatment until nine years later. We kept a close watch on my condition with frequent routine blood tests. Eventually, as expected, I resumed treatment, which has continued on and off over the years, with good results.

From my diagnosis in 1991 until March 2005, I kept my medical drama a secret. My caring wife and sister knew from the start about my problem. So did a very few others. These included my also caring assistant who has not only had to worry about me for the past 11 years, but also has had to transcribe all of my medical notes documenting my journey "for the file." I did not want other members of my family, including my mother and my children, to have to worry about me. I was not concerned (that much) because I knew I was receiving top care and remained optimistic about all that was in store.

However, I had to spill the beans in March 2005 when I was hospitalized because of pneumonia. While in the hospital, I was diagnosed with gastric and pulmonary amyloidosis (a rare complication that sometimes occurs in WM patients). I had been off medication at the time, but resumed chemotherapy, bringing the IgM antibody marker level that is used to track WM way down, successfully getting rid of the cause of the amyloid protein, a breakdown of the IgM antibody, that was in my lungs and gastrointestinal tract. By then, my secret was out. It had not been a strain on me to spare everyone regarding my condition; I took a mildly perverse pleasure in thinking that my disease was not serious enough to even make it evident to others. I was able to live a fairly normal life, without burdening too many people.

However, my partner in this, my wife (who has helped me through all of this, of course), was burdened with whatever there was to be burdened by, including my behavior which was sometimes influenced by steroids, a well-known side effect of these drugs. I first experienced the results of steroid medication early on in my treatment when I found myself cleaning the garage and moving household furniture at 2:00 in the morning— all resulting from my having received steroids that day. Also, once, after I responded entirely inappropriately to something she said, my wife ended up receiving (from me) a large gift certificate at her hairdresser's salon. I've tried to govern my behavior ever since, not only because she deserves better, but because of my budget limitations.

After the hospital visit, I was able to stop all treatment again when the IgM level became very low and there was no further concern regarding either the WM or associated amyloidosis.

I needed to resume treatment again in February 2012, when the gastric amyloidosis reappeared again. They disappeared in short order after a course of treatment with chemotherapy, steroids, and other drugs. Except for a three-month break from treatment most recently (and most recently resumed), I have been receiving every other week low doses of a medication called Velcade and steroids to keep the IgM level down and to avoid the development of more problems from the amyloidosis. Such has been successful. (In fact, my IgM level has recently reached 24-year lows, being either normal or close to it).

During all of these years, I continued to play handball, ski, bike, and backpack, needing to pick those times to do so when I was not troubled by a bit of anemia (such as it has been, on and off). Thankfully, I have not been anemic for quite a long time now. Also, I have worked full-time throughout my WM. We have been able to travel and live a mostly normal life. Although the reality of my condition has been a constant in my life from the start (when will something go wrong, or get worse), I have been thankful that all has gone as well as it has. For various reasons, much having to do with my running out of others to do certain things with, I have discontinued some of the above sports.

This year, I learned more about the further side effects from certain medications, e.g., prolonged steroid use can cause myopathy, which is a weakness in one's leg muscles. Such weakness can be addressed by regular exercise and other physical activities, all of which I am attempting to accomplish as soon as I get over a slight left hamstring pull I suffered last fall playing handball, and the right adductor strain suffered lifting weights at my local gym a few months ago. (I had quit handball about seven years ago, tried to start up again last fall, but have since quit again for various reasons unrelated to, but including, my physical condition.) As I have learned, these muscle injuries are contributed to by the myopathy, which also contributes to a delay in the muscle's ability to completely heal. I can say that this is the only problem relating to my condition which is affecting me now, and such is slowly resolving.

Since I wrote the above paragraph regarding myopathy, I've discovered that, perhaps, it was not caused by my treatment after all. I've more recently had a lumbar MRI prompted by a moderate radiculitis (pain extending down my legs), which became a problem a short time ago. I now have a new finding: a "severe" L4–L5 spinal stenosis that, no doubt, I've had all along but which only recently became evident and troublesome in its effects. It may be, therefore, that the muscle weakness has not been caused by the steroid treatment but instead by the stenosis. Either way, I'm responding with exercise and an anticipated epidural or two, as needed, in the future.

Now that I have shared my boring medical and personal history, let me talk about my un-boring relationship with Jim Berenson and all the people with or for whom (his patients) he works. First, let me say, again, how much I appreciate his caring, skill, thoughtfulness, compassion, knowledge, and sense of humor. I have greatly valued him as a person and as a doctor. Indeed, his reputation has been well earned. He is a well-known specialist dealing with my disease, as well as multiple myeloma, constantly speaking throughout the country. Over the years, I have benefitted from his state-of-the-art knowledge of these conditions. He has been "ahead of the game" in being able to prescribe the medicine I have needed and have benefitted from throughout.

Second, let me also say how much I appreciate the kindness and caring expressed by everybody that works with him and for him at his clinic.

Third, let me use the word "family" to describe all of my fellow patients (and nurses). I cannot say that I look forward to getting treatment at the clinic (although I do, considering its value and necessity), but let me say that I otherwise look forward to spending time with all those people I see every two weeks (or as necessary) sitting around with needles stuck in their arms receiving treatment. We support each other, laugh, talk seriously, and share much. Dr. Berenson's staff is concerned about us, and we are all concerned about each other. It is easier for me to accept what I must go through when I am sitting with others who are having the same experience and enduring the same challenges. Perhaps the most important contribution I make to the sharing process is when I bring cookies to the treatment room (as do others) on those days when I must spend some time there. We pass around the snacks and keep everyone nourished. The nurses are careful not to take more than their share (I think)—just kidding. To the contrary, I don't see them eating enough of the cookies.

What keeps me going (and, I am sure, everyone else) is the realization that Dr. Berenson's research is continuing even as we sit there receiving medication. Not only is it comforting to know that I am among friends, my fellow patients, but I am in the company of a friend, Dr. Jim Berenson, upon whom I can rely to do his best for me while he continues his search for a cure for our diseases.

My Waldenstrom's is considered incurable but treatable. From the beginning, I had confidence that things would work out, and they have. I have come to consider my disease as merely "a nuisance," one needing thoughtful attention and a lot of time, but...so what.

We patients have been able to share our successes, problems, and discomfort with each other. We are not alone, we have each other and we have our spouses, partners, family, and friends. Most important, we have Dr. Jim Berenson, Regina, Barbara, the nurses, and everyone else at the clinic. We are all in this together. Thank you all.

I Have WHAT???

By Bradley K. -- MGUS?!!

Age: 50

Music Composer and Real Estate Investor

It all began on Monday, April 26, 2004 at 10:00 a.m. when I went in for a routine annual physical exam. There was nothing atypical about this particular physical. I felt perfectly fine, as always, and had the usual breezy chat with my internist. Two days later I was diagnosed with a monoclonal protein spike, and on May 7, 2004 I learned more about this particular M-protein. That was more than 11 years ago. While I continue to exhibit good physical health, I live with the awareness that I harbor a monoclonal protein that remains at a level low enough to be of "underdetermined significance," and I'm told it is very likely here to stay.

"You have MGUS," said the internist. "MGUS," I mouthed to myself. A benign-sounding acronym. Aside from the "M" part, "Gus" is a common nickname—casual, nonthreatening. For some reason, I thought about the former astronaut, Gus Grissom. He was brave. He had the right stuff. Suffice it to say, the acronym "MGUS" didn't register with me. In fact, I wasn't alone. Many physicians don't recognize the acronym, but they do understand the meaning of Monoclonal Gammopathy of Undetermined Significance.

Aside from an asymptomatic diagnosis of osteoporosis and osteopenia for which I receive biannual Zometa infusions, there have been no other physical reminders of my disease since I was first diagnosed at age 41. Still, the test results continue to remind me that I have something. In addition to "MGUS," other medical acronyms like SPEP, UPEP, and IFE have become a familiar part of my lexicon. Dr. Berenson recently added another test to the mix, called the Serum Free Light Chain Assay (SFLCA). My SFLCA test results show some extra abnormalities that, according to Dr. Berenson, put me at a somewhat higher risk, but not by very much. As is my wont, I spent hours researching free light chains. While my own research seemed to indicate a higher risk than what Dr. Berenson conveyed, I am drawn to the comforting humor of Mark Twain who said, "I am an old man and have known a great many troubles, but most of them never happened."

Perhaps this diagnosis is like a "kick in the pants," a reminder that life is, indeed, not a dress rehearsal. It's the "now" that counts—the music I am composing now, the people in my life now, the places I am traveling to now, the literature I am reading now and, yes, even the things I am learning about my disease now. The human body is like an inner universe, as much a frontier as our outer universe. I see Dr. Berenson as the captain of this particular exploration and we, his patients, are part of the crew. In an odd way, perhaps it's the quest itself—the quest for understanding, the quest for cures—that makes life worth living.

I Have WHAT???

By Dale H. -- MULTIPLE MYELOMA?!!

Age: Late 70s

Writer

Sailing along, confident in the knowledge I was going to live forever, (half of my high school graduating class had already passed away—but not me), and why not? The planet has been here for over a billion years. I was made of the same stuff as the planet, and at age 72 and in perfect health I was heading for a major surf trip to El Salvador. All I needed was a few vaccinations against hepatitis B and hepatitis C, as the sanitation there is not the greatest and the places where I like to surf are the point breaks off river mouths where the sewage usually flows down to the sea. I felt great, and going in to get the shots from my primary care doc he took the usual blood tests and—whoops, slow down—when the result came in he called me and said, "You're anemic."

I said, "That's okay." I said, "I'll just take some iron."

"No," he said, "that's not it. There's a problem with your blood work."

"Oh? No big deal. I'll just get in better shape."

"No," he answers, "your sed rate is very high. It's over 100."

The brush of the angel's wings across your face as you sleep.

When I told my wife, who knew what that meant, she gasped.

The diagnosis comes and it's multiple myeloma, a cancer of the blood. It's incurable, and fatal.

Now it's the Devil's tail slapping you directly in the face as you stare at him, wide awake.

"I have a doctor I recommend for you," my PC doc said.

We all know we are going to die, but we don't know when and we don't know how.

Those mysteries now start narrowing down.

The educational reading begins.

The visits to the different doctors. The X-rays, bone scans, and bone marrow biopsy.

Recommended Doctor Number One was decent. He said, "You do have MM. It's in a smoldering stage right now, but that could change at any moment. I can treat you, but for your own peace of mind you should get another opinion. Do that and then come back."

The next doctor was at UCLA. He was a nice man with a wall full of framed degrees and pictures he'd taken of Arctic animals, mostly penguins. He quickly decided that it was best to attack the MM right away.

We asked: "How long can one smolder, before treatment is absolutely called for?"

The answer was, "No one knows."

"Then I could smolder indefinitely, and perhaps die of something else?"

"It's best to treat you now," he repeated.

Doctor Number Three was back east at Harvard.

My wife's best friend had a rare condition called amyloidosis and was treated by this doctor. He got her into remission. His specialty, however, was MM. This was where he had his best results and was the most acclaimed.

So, my wife, Deborah, and I made an appointment, which luckily enough was the only one he had open for several months, and we flew to Boston.

We waited for three hours, and finally the great man takes us into his office. We find ourselves in a room with him, along with two other doctors, one who has come from Italy and the other from Israel to study under him.

Seating us off to the side, he conducts the exam speaking about me only in the third person, never talking directly to us, never making eye contact, talking only to the other doctors.

His purpose is to impress them with the superiority of his personal diagnostic techniques.

Suddenly, in mid-interview, he downgrades my smoldering state to full-on active myeloma, according to him, and I'm in need of immediate treatment.

Now it's the Devil slamming the three-pronged pitchfork directly into your heart.

The examination over, he tells me to go outside the room and see the nurse, who will draw some additional blood, which he will forward on to Cedars-Sinai back in Los Angeles where I will immediately start treatment upon our return.

This only takes a few minutes. Deborah and I leave and go toward the elevator to go down to the street. Both of us are, as you no doubt already know, stunned, devastated, and completely numb all at the same time.

Then, just as the elevator doors almost close, a hand from outside reaches between the doors and stops the action. The woman doctor from Israel steps in. We think she is going down with us.

She looks at me, then at Deborah, then back at me, and carefully shakes her head, "No," while putting her finger up to her lips, smiling behind the warning to stay silent about what she has just let us know, and steps back and exits.

The doors close, and Deborah and I both go, "Wow."

Her implication is absolutely clear: Please go see someone else.

That someone else turned out to be Doctor Berenson. No talking down. No rush to judgment. A careful monitoring schedule set up. Zometa was what he recommended, and that was all that I received to treat my myeloma.

Dr. Berenson put me on a monthly dose and checked my labs. For three years, I led a somewhat normal life, albeit one full of anxiety. Then I had what seemed like a kidney stone attack. My markers spiked and Dr. Berenson said it was time for treatment, a combination of Doxil, Dex, and Velcade.

The odd thing is that the treatment, which I had so dreaded, was less anxiety-provoking than waiting for the pitchfork to slam into my heart again.

And the treatment quickly reduced my numbers and put me into remission.

I am currently on a maintenance treatment consisting of Dex and Velcade, administered once every two weeks in clinic, and oral Medrol, taken every other day. I am entering my ninth month of this without any myeloma showing itself in my blood or urine.

None of this really matters to you who are reading this. Each of us who will get MM, or have it, will have a similar story, unique and personal in its details, but forcing one to face the facts and try to find the best way to deal with its reality.

I only now want to tell you what I have learned that may be of help to you, the reader.

Get an ally. Whether this is a wife, husband, lover, relative, a friend, or even if you need to hire someone, MM is an emotional journey and one to be undertaken with clarity of mind. When you are newly operating under a death sentence and trying to figure a way out, chances are you won't be thinking objectively. Someone else who is not in your body, sitting and listening, may hear things entirely differently than you do.

In my own case, my tendency is to try to make the doctor like me, so he or she will give me their best attention and medical care. Often, I am so busy doing this I don't actually hear (or don't want to hear) what the doctor is clearly stating. I leave the exam room not remembering what I was told.

In other words, I am at times my own worst enemy.

I've been lucky. And I mean really lucky. My wife is objective. She listens and listens accurately. So much so that Dr. B calls her Dr. Deborah.

Which brings me to Dr. B.

Thank you, Jim.

I Have WHAT???

By Gene B. -- MULTIPLE MYELOMA?!!

Age: 60s

Real Estate and Mortgage Broker

That one might learn the true meaning of the word *serendipity* when the stakes are the highest is indeed an incredible blessing.

On April 13 (a Friday, no less), 2007, I was admitted to the local hospital, needing a transfusion of six units of blood and an immediate dialysis treatment (having been without kidney function for some time—the test results indicated for over a week). My lab numbers were so upside down, the admitting nurse, in a conversation several weeks later, told my wife and I that no one had expected me to live for even 24 hours. When, after my transfusion and dialysis treatment, I was taken to my room in the hospital for what would ultimately be an eight-day stay, I was greeted by my wife, Enid, and a physician from the internal medicine practice (who had, with some considerable effort, totally bungled what might have been an earlier, and more beneficial to me, diagnosis of my illness). Both of them sat at my bedside—my wife with an anxious look and the physician with both hands showing crossed fingers.

That doctor's first words: "We'll know in 24 hours." I asked what we would know. He answered, "Whether you'll live or not." He then went on to inform me that I had "multiple myeloma." Two words at that moment meant nothing to me, as I had no idea of this disease to which they related. He apparently could see that in my expression. So he elaborated, "Blood cancer." I knew those words. And I knew even more that this could not be good.

An hour or so later, *Serendipitous Event #1*: Another physician came into my room and introduced himself as the on-call oncologist. He explained to Enid and me, now both totally in shock after learning my diagnosis, the nature of this heretofore (to us, at least) unknown illness. We then discussed how he recommended my treatments should ensue. He suggested that we commence with what was considered to be the standard frontline drug at that time to treat multiple myeloma, thalidomide, and have radiation treatments to prevent further spinal damage from the compression fractures of the thoracic spine at T10, T11, and T12 that I presented with at the time of my admission to the hospital.

On my second day, after having a second dialysis procedure and initial plasmapheresis treatment (to try to get rid of the proteins that were causing my kidneys to not work), I was transferred by ambulance across the street to the radiation treatment center. There, I would be tattooed to mark the sites for the radiation treatments that were to begin the following day at approximately 4:00 p.m. So for most of my first two days in the hospital, I was tethered to large, whirring machines whose function I could only guess, but were aimed at saving my life.

On Day 3, *Serendipitous Event #2*: Our oncologist shared that although he treats many patients in his practice with multiple myeloma, he did not at all consider himself an expert on this illness. For that reason, he shared two names with us. The first was the head of the myeloma section of the hematology-oncology department at UCSF. The second, he said, is a somewhat unconventional practitioner, Dr. James Berenson, whose Los Angeles-based oncology practice solely deals with multiple myeloma. In that we are residents of Northern California, and with the excellent reputation of UCSF, it seemed only logical that we first attempt to contact the UCSF reference. Which Enid did, as soon as the oncologist left my room? After numerous switchboard redirections, she reached the office of the doctor we were seeking. Enid was told that this doctor was away on vacation, and would not return to the hospital for another ten days (*Serendipitous Event #3*).

That left us with the choice of waiting for him to return or to try to reach Dr. James Berenson. Given our high level of anxiety and hunger for more information, I called Dr. Berenson's office and was greeted by a lady named Barbara (*Serendipitous Event #4*). I briefly described the reason for my call. Barbara gave me Dr. Berenson's cell phone number (imagine my surprise at that) and suggested that I call him directly. I did just that immediately after concluding my conversation with Barbara. Dr. Berenson answered the phone, and I explained how I had been given his direct phone number. He interrupted and told me he was with a patient and would have to call me later that afternoon. I gave him my cell number. In my heart, I hoped I'd hear back from him. In my head, all I heard was, "Sure, he's not really going to call me back!"

As I was scheduled for my first radiation treatment at 4:00 p.m. that day, at approximately 3:15 p.m., I was changing into pajamas to keep my derrière from being exposed during the transfer back across the street to the radiation treatment center for my first radiation treatment. My cell phone rang (from a timing standpoint, for reasons that will become clear below, this was *Serendipitous Event #5*). To my great surprise, Dr. Berenson introduced himself on the other end of the line. He said, "Tell me what's going on with you." I proceeded to give him a Cliff's notes version of my sordid history of misdiagnosis, current medical status (zero kidney function, three compression fractures, upside down lab values, etc.), hospitalization, and treatment plan, especially the then-pending pickup by the ambulance drivers for my initial radiation treatment. Without any hesitation, Dr. Berenson suggested that if I could stand the back pain for another couple of weeks, he'd strongly recommend that I should not undergo the radiation treatments. He told me there was a new procedure being done. He could refer me to an orthopedic surgeon who could perform a procedure called a balloon kyphoplasty, that would not only resolve my back pain, but also not obliterate the chief remaining (at my age) bone marrow-producing areas of my body in the spine and pelvic region, which would occur if I proceeded with the planned radiation treatments that were supposed to begin at that very moment. He went on to explain that I'd need that bone marrow production in the long run to be able to tolerate future treatments that I would require. This seemed totally logical and it started my deep affinity for a man who, over time, I came to learn was not only logical, but extremely smart about myeloma. Dr. Berenson is totally devoted to patients enjoying the best quality of life possible with this unfortunate diagnosis.

At just about that point in our conversation, the ambulance people appeared at my hospital room door. It took them totally by surprise when, while still on the phone with Dr. Berenson, I sent them away and told them I was not going for the "ride" that afternoon.

As we concluded our conversation, Dr. Berenson suggested I call and make an appointment to see him after I was discharged from the hospital, as soon as I felt I could handle a plane trip to Southern California.

A few hours later, the radiation therapy doctor who had prescribed the treatments appeared in my hospital room doorway. He asked why I had refused treatment #1. I explained that I had received and decided to follow a second opinion to delay the start of this regimen (I dared not say it had been suggested over the phone, for fear of being committed for a psychiatric evaluation), but I would let him know when I decided it was time to commence the radiation therapy. (Like as in *never*!)

Enid's and my trip to Los Angeles occurred approximately two weeks after my hospital discharge. During those two weeks, I was receiving dialysis three times a week. The thalidomide that I was taking unfortunately quickly caused blood clotting in my right jugular vein (which to this day, almost six years later, is totally clotted), down to the toes of my right foot. And as a result, my right calf and ankle were swollen to a size one and a half times larger than my left. I also lost total control of my right foot. Enid called me Flipper. To walk at all, I needed a cane (for which I selected a five-iron from my golf bag--I did not want to be seen moving about with a real cane). This was now due less to the back pain but more to the neurologic and vascular damage caused by the drug being used to treat my myeloma, thalidomide. I later learned from Dr. Berenson that that might have been obviated to some degree had blood-thinning measures commenced as soon as the thalidomide pills had first been taken by me. But, even in that somewhat incapacitated state, I considered myself to be as travel-ready as I might ever be.

Finally, we arrived at what I soon would understand is the Mecca for those of us unfortunate enough to be diagnosed with multiple myeloma, which is where Enid and I met Dr. Berenson (*the 6th and most important of the Serendipitous Events in this chronology*). We were "armed" with what we thought were the right questions to ask. Like: "In what stage is my illness?" Dr. Berenson's mouth curled into a half-smile and repeated, with a questioning tone, the word, "Stage?" He continued: "Your kidneys are gone, your back is broken, and your lab numbers are upside down…I'd say you're in the *suck* stage." That one-liner was the most important single comment made by this man, who I then knew for only ten minutes. It told me that I would never have to guess what he was thinking. And neither was he one to sugarcoat the facts.

He went on to suggest that the thalidomide treatment regimen I was on should be immediately changed to what was then not considered standard frontline therapy. He prescribed a three-drug combination of dexamethasone, Velcade, and Doxil (DVD) that he had developed from his laboratory work and was highly successful in clinical studies that he was conducting to treat myeloma. He also explained that if my kidneys had any possibility of returning to function, this regimen (and not thalidomide) would give me the best chance. He further explained that this would likely take approximately six to eight weeks to occur.

This was the beginning of (at the time of this writing) a seven-year relationship, which has seen the following occur by the total *serendipity* of our becoming acquainted with Dr. James Berenson, and now having his hands, together with a very smart and compassionate local oncologist, guiding my treatment during this entire time.

Week 5 after diagnosis, I received the balloon kyphoplasty procedure to fix my collapsed vertebral bodies in my spine. I entered the hospital unable to walk upright and only ambulatory with the use of my five-iron "cane." I left the hospital 25 hours later walking upright and with no need for any aid! I was playing golf (even if not quite as well as before being diagnosed with myeloma) six weeks after the surgery.

Week 6 after diagnosis and Week 3 after beginning on the DVD regimen, I received a call from my nephrologist, advising she had good news—there were some signs of return of my kidney function, and that I could reduce my dialysis regimen to two times per week.

Week 7, another "good news" call from the nephrologist, which I thought would be to advise that I might be cut down to once a week. Instead she advised I would no longer need dialysis—that adequate kidney function had returned to eliminate the need for it to continue. As anyone familiar with the rigors of dialysis knows, this was huge in advancing my quality of life and my desire to go on living.

Lovenox treatments commenced to try to resolve the blood clots; shortly thereafter, through today, both my calves and ankles became the same size and my right foot became totally functional again.

In the ensuing 14 months, the DVD regimen had brought my myeloma blood tests, my IgG, and M-protein levels down to a somewhat manageable level. This then enabled the collection of stem cells for a hypothetical future transplant, which, as anyone in Dr. Berenson's care intimately knows, he would not recommend until/unless all other options (which he now describes as nearly an endless choice of treatments) had failed.

At that point, when there were signs that the hold this DVD drug regimen had on the myeloma was losing its grip and the disease was worsening, came *Serendipitous Event #7*: The almost simultaneous FDA approval for clinical use of the successor drug to thalidomide called Revlimid. Since then, for approximately the past four years, at Dr. Berenson's direction, I have been on a low dose of this drug and a few others to the amazing effect of a near-zero M-spike level, normal (if not, often, even low) IgG levels, and normal free kappa and lambda light chain levels and associated ratios in my blood.

In the ensuing years, while undergoing the most current regimen, there is now movement by other thought leaders in his field toward concurrence with Dr. Berenson's view that stem cell transplantation is not for everyone, and may not even be good for anyone as a primary therapy.

For the past three years, I have participated as a proud board member of IMBCR, and as one of its most avid fundraisers, to keep the fires burning brightly at this amazing Institute.

Today, my full-time work as a real estate and loan broker is completely unimpeded by the near totally oral regimen I am on to keep hold on the myeloma—the only exception is a monthly infusion of a bone strengthener called Zometa (very small price) that Dr. Berenson actually gave to the first patient in the world back in 1995. In spite of the anemia that comes with Revlimid treatment, I exercise regularly. I ride my road bike (most notably on a 70-mile, 6-hour trek to raise money for Dr. Berenson's IMBCR). I play golf, something I never thought would be in my future had I not undergone kyphoplasty as Dr. Berenson had recommended and explained to me and my wife on the phone. I travel with my wife and our two Standard Poodles on extended RV trips across the United States. I teach real estate at the local Junior College. I live a virtually normal life.

What is more important and quite simply stated, I *live* with a quality of life I never thought possible as a blood cancer patient. I tell people who know of my diagnosis, "If I did not know I was sick, I would not think I was sick." Absolutely none of this would have been even remotely possible had the true meaning of the word *serendipity* not been vividly shown to me by one of the most caring, and to my way of thinking, the most knowledgeable practitioner in this ever-changing field—much of the dynamic of which is driven by the tireless efforts of one man: Dr. James Berenson, and the Institute for Myeloma & Bone Cancer Research which he founded more than a decade ago.

I Have WHAT???

By Geoff W. -- MULTIPLE MYELOMA?!!

Age: 50ish

Investment Manager

I did all the right things…ate oatmeal every day, biked, skied, and had an active lifestyle. Like many aging baby boomers, at 50, I was planning to live forever. Needless to say, getting diagnosed with multiple myeloma was a bolt out of the blue. It was September 2006, and I was trying my hand at wakeboarding near Park City, Utah. At my family's and friend's insistence, I rounded the lake again, but this time I collided with the wake and came up out of the water howling as my shoulder broke on impact.

Initially, I made the mistake of researching MM on the internet, only to find grim mortality statistics that I later found were obsolete. I explored treatment options, including stem cell transplantation. Fortunately for me, I had a neighbor in oncology that steered me to Dr. Berenson. From the moment I met with "Dr. B" in the "Alta room" (all of his exam rooms are named after ski areas—Alta is one of my favorite ski areas in Utah and I later learned Dr. Berenson's very favorite one), I knew I had found a doctor I could relate to. Dr.

Berenson offered me genuine hope as he described numerous treatment options, and the improved longevity of his patients, who were living far longer than the statistics I had read.

My MM Journey

After a few weeks of self-pity and fear of the unknown, I decided that if I had less time, I wasn't going to waste it. After a number of treatment cycles, I realized that while the chemo took me at times from my usual 110% down to 80%, Dr. B was committed to helping his patients maintain their normal lifestyle. He and his staff closely monitored not just the “numbers,” but also how the disease and treatments were affecting my energy level and activities. My lifestyle pre-MM consisted of demanding work as an investment manager, some 20-plus days a year of skiing, frequent travel, and best of all, a fulfilling life as husband and father of my then twin nine-year olds. Remarkably, post-MM, under Dr. B’s astute care, my lifestyle hasn't changed; something I never would have even dreamed was possible when I was first diagnosed. What has changed is that I am much more aware that life is short and how important it is to live in the now.

During my six years since diagnosis, I have been treated with various “cocktails,” with long periods of “maintenance” in between. These treatments have included various trials of which Dr. B has been at the forefront, as he translates his laboratory work at the Institute for Myeloma & Bone Cancer Research into clinical trials. Having a doctor who can quickly recognize whether a regimen is working, determine how long to treat, and adjust dosages to the patient's unique physiology and psychology is critical. Better yet, Dr. Berenson's warmth, concern, and humor make it all go down easier.

While treatments certainly take a toll, I have found that an active regimen of exercise helps me combat the side effects and fatigue. In 2009, I embarked on an odyssey of treks with a group of like-minded friends. We hiked to the top of Yosemite's Half Dome, and followed this with an unforgettable trek along the Inca Trail to the mysterious Machu Picchu. In 2010, we summited Mount Whitney in a day (the hardest physical ordeal I have ever faced—over 17 hours). This was a "training hike" culminating that summer with our ascent to the top of Mount Kilimanjaro, Africa's highest mountain at 19,341 feet. After four years, I was still going strong. I expressed my gratitude to Dr. B and his staff in a summit photo with my wife, which is on display in his clinic and featured in a cancer magazine. Not only was Dr. Berenson flexible with my treatment regimen so I could pursue these goals, he even introduced me to a fellow patient and doctor who had traveled to over 100 countries. He was able to advise me on the vaccinations required as I ventured into South America and Africa!

So what has changed for me?

Well, for one, I have a new friend that I ski with—Dr. Berenson, who is an expert skier. However, two seasons ago, my wife and I put Dr. B through the ropes at *our* favorite ski area in Utah, The

Canyons. Regrettably, he took a bad fall on a double black diamond run we led him down that had insufficient snow, and he commented at the time, "I need a free consult from your wife" (who happens to be an orthopedist). When I returned to the office, I was admonished not to "kill our doctor!"

Every month, I look forward to getting my next "report card" with my M-spike or "myeloma numbers" to see how well the latest treatment is working. The news has been good most of the time. But when the news isn't so good, often I get a call from Dr. B ahead of my visit. This helps me prepare mentally and gives my wife and I time to consider other treatment options. My wife has also been an incredible support as she spends hours researching the latest studies and findings. Dr. B patiently answers questions, sometimes offering other treatment options if appropriate.

Also, I have made new friends at Dr. B's office. We cover the gamut of topics, as well as compare notes on our latest treatments. All the while, we are cared for by Dr. B's wonderful nursing and professional staff. In addition, I have a new "second office" there, where I read, take work calls, and catch up on my investment reading.

Most of all, MM has given me determination to live life to its fullest. While I'm not ready for retirement, at six years and counting, I realize MM will take its toll, and so I have a fierce desire to refocus on my "bucket list." I have started a four-day workweek and look forward to more "me" time, as well as more time with my wife and children who will soon be graduating from high school. I now look forward to seeing them graduate from college, too, and perhaps even get married, which is a gift I could never have imagined six years ago, all because of the help from my doctor—and fellow skier!

I Have WHAT???

By Jack B. -- MULTIPLE MYELOMA?!!

Age: 60's

Business Owner

I was diagnosed with multiple myeloma more than 6 years ago and at the time it came as a shock. I was not feeling sick and other than having lower back pain, I was not aware than anything was wrong. Occasionally I would fall or "trip" but I blamed it on my bad knees and rolled-up carpet. Eventually it turned out that the bad back pain was really a severe compression of the spinal cord which was also responsible for my falls.

The initial diagnosis of the disease with the awful "C" was devastating for my close family members and me! My initial reaction was that this was a life sentence and that it surely meant that death was near. I remember making pronouncements to my family and close friends as if it was the last time that they would ever hear me speak to them.

The oncologist that we first saw was very nice person but his prognosis for my multiple myeloma was not great. My son later told me that when he asked that same oncologist how many other patients he had treated with this condition, he said he had treated only a few over the years because it was a very rare cancer.

During this initial diagnosis period, I was completely unable to make decisions about my own care so I asked my two sons who were in their 30's to help me. As a business owner, I am usually the one in charge and I like to make decisions. But, as anyone who gets a similar diagnosis knows-- you're not in the best place to make decisions. One of my sons called a few friends who were doctors and asked them about oncologists that specialize in multiple myeloma. Luckily for me, one of the doctors he called had a wife who was also a medical professional. She had been an intern for Dr. Berenson. She spoke very highly of him and his level of research and knowledge in the area.

Just to be certain, my son also arranged a consultation with City of Hope; the doctor we met was very nice but the solution he discussed centered on transplant. I do remember an incident, which now makes me laugh. I asked the doctor at City of Hope how long I was going to live and his response was "only God knows exactly when you will die." From that conversation, I only heard "you will die" which goes to show you definitely need a family member to go with you to these initial consultations -- because it's just so overwhelming.

Our next stop was Dr. Berenson's office, and he was immediately reassuring. He was clear that he knew how to treat myeloma and that his approach was to use the latest technology and medicine to treat the disease. It was like you would treat diabetes -- something that you need to treat but that otherwise you can continue living your life.

We felt comfortable with Dr. Berenson and I immediately became his patient. My sons could resume their lives and stop doing independent Google research regarding my disease. We could all be comfortable that the day a new technology or medicine became available not only would Dr. B know about it but more than likely he was going to be speaking on the subject or be doing additional research on it or maybe he even had a hand in its discovery and development.

In my personal opinion, to make it through this type of disease you need have faith in a higher power, the support of family and friends and a good doctor to be as dedicated as Dr. Berenson is to treat patients with this disease. What I love about Dr. Berenson is that if he sees even a slight change for the worse, he is already thinking about how to adjust the treatment. I feel confident that Dr. Berenson is as concerned about my health as any family member would be. He is laser focused on keeping his patients healthy so that they can live the most satisfying lives possible.

I Have WHAT???

By Jackie R. -- MULTIPLE MYELOMA?!!

Age: 48

Therapist

Receiving a cancer diagnosis is like falling down a rabbit hole or being abducted by aliens. It is surreal. A parallel universe. From the minute Dr. Berenson told me I had cancer, everything felt different. Ambient laughter felt abrasive, sunshine felt harsh, music made me cry. All I knew to be true in my life had changed in a moment. But although I didn't feel it at the time, there was still hope. There is always hope.

At the time of my diagnosis, almost three years ago, I was 45 years old, married, with an 11-year old daughter. Ironically, I had recently received a Master's degree in psychology and was gaining my clinical experience at The Cancer Support Community (formerly The Wellness Community) as a therapist-intern, co-facilitating cancer support groups. I am so grateful for my pre-diagnosis time at the Cancer Support Community—a crash course in how to navigate the world I was dropped into. What I learned there, and continue to learn, has been invaluable to my success at living my life with cancer.

I strongly encourage anyone with cancer to join a support group—there is nothing like being with people who really "get it" to combat the feeling of loneliness that cancer patients often experience.

Telling people "I have cancer" is extremely difficult—saying the words makes it real, and you are forever changing the way people see you. Some people show up for you in ways you would never expect, while others disappear. I choose to believe people do their best, and I welcome the love I receive from those who are present rather than resent those who find the situation too difficult.

It took me a while to believe I had cancer. An oncologist six months prior had misdiagnosed me, and when Dr. Berenson told me I had multiple myeloma I was sure he was mistaken. No matter how many times and in how many ways he said my cells were malignant, it wasn't registering. I was experiencing everyone's worst nightmare. Films, television, and novels—the person with cancer usually ends up dead. I denied it for as long as possible, all the while moving forward with what needed to be done, as if I were humoring everyone while waiting for the call that would confirm my belief that it was all a big mistake. Unfortunately, that call never came.

The beginning was the worst, like being swept up in a tsunami. The learning curve was huge, the doctor appointments, scans, and tests were endless, and the scary questions—"How will I care for my daughter?"; "How sick will I get?"; "Will my health insurance pay for my treatment?" and of course, the big one, "How long will I live?"—

filled my day and plagued my mind. Even as I received my first chemo treatment, through a port-a-cath that had been inserted surgically into my chest, I still felt it was all a frightful mistake. Most likely for self-preservation, my mind was unable to accept the reality of my diagnosis. Eventually, however, the truth leaks in.

The most important piece of advice I would want to impart to any newly diagnosed patient is to get more than one opinion and see an oncologist who specializes in your specific type of cancer. I can't imagine going through this challenging experience without a doctor I trust and respect both personally and professionally, and am so incredibly grateful I found my way to Dr. Berenson. When I started my treatments, I would talk to my fellow patients as we were all hooked up to our chemo bags. Over and over I heard endless stories about how extraordinary Dr. Berenson is. While it was a great comfort to hear such high praise for the person whom I had just handed my life over to, to be perfectly honest, the admiration seemed extreme. I joked that Dr. Berenson must be giving everyone the "Kool-Aid" in their chemo bags (a reference to the Jonestown cult where the members blindly followed their leader). I soon realized, however, that their loyalty and love towards Dr. B wasn't because he was spiking their IVs, it was because he is passionate about what he does and knows everything there is to know about the cancer he treats. And most importantly, he believes, as I do, that he will find a cure for this cancer.

But that's just the medical side of Dr. B. The human side is that he isn't afraid to develop friendships with his patients. For me, feeling comfortable with my doctor, feeling a connection, gives me more power over my cancer. Having a disease can make you feel "less-than," which contributes to the loss of control and loss of hope so many patients experience, but the actions of a compassionate doctor can help lessen these feelings of despair. Dr. B makes the day-to-day minutiae of dealing with cancer less stressful. Giving me his cell phone number so I never feel abandoned, having machines in his office that allow blood tests to be run onsite, having an arsenal of competent doctors for referrals all alleviates stress. In addition, his approach of honesty coated with optimism helps me move forward, hopeful each day.

Early on in my diagnosis, I brought my daughter to one of my treatments, hoping the reality of chemo would be less scary for her than whatever images she was conjuring in her mind. I was confident that Barbara, the first voice on the phone when you call the office and the first face you see when you arrive, would ease my girl's anxiety just as she does for every patient and family member who walks through the door. The importance of this first contact should not be underestimated. I remember on the day of my initial appointment, Barbara, probably reading the fear in my face, said to me, "Whatever you find out today, you are in the best place you could be." And I believed her. I also trusted that Dr. Berenson would have some words of wisdom for my daughter, and a dad himself, he was able to answer questions and quell fears. I was confident that the kind nurses and the upbeat atmosphere would help soothe my daughter's worries. After spending a couple of hours in the office, watching me get vitals taken, blood drawn, and treatment administered, she said, "I think I want to be a doctor like Regina" (referring to the head nurse). I informed her that Regina was a nurse and Dr. Berenson was the doctor. She contemplated this for a while, and then said that she thought being a nurse might be more interesting than being a doctor because "nurses actually get to do stuff" other than "walk back and forth like Dr. Berenson, which seems like it would get boring." Thank God for great nurses.

My strongest advice to the newly diagnosed (after finding the best doctor) is to trust your instinct. Many well-intentioned family members and friends will fill your in-box with cures, healers, do's and don'ts, articles, sage opinions as well as ill-advised ideas. Read what you want, delete what you don't. Some patients are researchers, some aren't. Personally, I like to do as much research as I can, usually on the internet. Information gives me power. For some people, it is too scary, and that's okay. Once you have gathered the information you feel you need, go with what resonates for you. What works for one person, whether it is a certain treatment, a diet, an exercise regime, or an attitude, might not work for someone else. Our instincts can carry us far if we let them. That said…here's *my* well-intentioned advice regarding diet. I have been following The Budwig Diet for two years, along with my treatment. I believe the reason I have been able to stay on maintenance treatment for so long (after responding to my initial treatment as part of a five-month clinical trial) is because of this diet.

The science behind it makes sense—it has even sparked Dr. Berenson's interest. I strongly urge anyone with cancer to research this diet and give it a try.

There are some cancer patients who view their illness as a gift—I am *not* one of them. However, I do believe that I have control over how I react to the challenges this disease has presented in my life. And how I choose to react is my power. No matter what challenges I face, it is the *reaction* to the challenge that dictates the course of my life. As for being *positive*, that too is interpretive and doesn't mean I can't be sad, angry, or just exhausted, in addition to being *hopeful*. They are not mutually exclusive feelings! While I wrestle the esoteric concerns that come with a life-threatening illness, it is heartening to know that I am not in this alone. I am filled with gratitude, not only for Dr. B and his staff, but for my loving family and friends, for my co-patients alongside me in the foxhole, and, mostly, for all those multiple myeloma patients who came and went before me, and whose disease helped move research forward so all of us could live longer, more satisfying lives with myeloma.

I Have WHAT???

By James T., MD -- MULTIPLE MYELOMA?!!

Age: 60s

Endocrinologist

Dr. T. was a founding board member of the Institute for Myeloma & Bone Cancer Research (IMBCR). He was also a patient of Dr. Berenson's. He fought this disease for more than ten years and acknowledged that this was due in great part to the dedication of Dr. Berenson and his research. These are the words he chose to write:

Dr. Berenson is probably the foremost expert on this disease in America. This is for several reasons:

First, he is a doctor's doctor; namely, he directs intensive bench science research while, at the same time, still participates in the front lines of seeing patients. This makes him unique. He can see a patient in the office, obtain a bone marrow sample, and simply walk across the hall to the Institute's state of the art research laboratory. Within minutes a process starts that can take that individual's bone marrow into an analysis in which he will attempt to see which therapy is most appropriate. This rapid sequence has obviously helped give new life to me and to other patients.

Second, Dr. Berenson has such a broad knowledge of the field of myeloma and bone cancer that when he says something isn't working, he knows where to go next. He helped me over the years modify my treatments with the newer agents as they became available. I sometimes envisioned myself as a surfer, riding and balancing the crest of the waves that have the potential to take me under water. I saw Dr. Berenson as my surfing instructor keeping me on top.

Dr. T. was a resident of Palos Verdes and Clinical Associate Professor of Medicine at UCLA Medical Center. He maintained an active medical practice in Redondo Beach for more than 23 years.

I Have WHAT???

By Jay C. -- MULTIPLE MYELOMA?!!

Age: 75

Former Los Angeles Laker

A Little Myeloma Humor…

I had my first brush with the "C-word" 25 years ago. I felt a mass in my right pectoral. My breast was removed and the tumor turned out to be benign. The surgeon was a lady feminist. I could tell because she sewed my nipple on crooked just to get even. I've been kinda scared walking on the beaches in Santa Barbara ever since.

Fifteen years later the scare was for real. I had prostate cancer. I chose treatment with protons in Loma Linda, California. We rented a condo in Palm Springs for two months and I commuted an hour each way for my 45 treatments. We made a vacation out of it. It was memorable because they encouraged us to have as much sex as we could stand. They wanted my prostate gland to be as active as possible. The treatment worked and I didn't have any of the three side effects patients often get from other forms of treatment. I don't pee when I sneeze. I don't have to wear diapers for the other end either. And I don't need blue pills. I had six months of sweats between testing for a couple of years, but all in all, prostate cancer ended up being a happy memory. I know that sounds strange but that's the way it was for me. It must have been all the sex.

Five years ago, everything changed. We were living in Maui and I came down with pneumonia. Through a routine blood test the medical lab discovered I had myeloma. "I have what?" I asked. And the medical person said I couldn't see an oncologist for three weeks. I looked at the mortality rates and discovered I had two and a half years to live. Don't tell me I have an incurable cancer and I'll have to wait three weeks to do anything about it. That wasn't going to fly.

Maui is not a good place to get sick. The medical system isn't very good. They told me on Good Friday. We flew back to Santa Barbara on Saturday and saw an oncologist on Monday. The doctor gave me Zometa (a bone hardening drug) without checking to see if I needed it. His nurse wasn't there so he stuck the needle in for the infusion. Never let a doctor do that to you. They don't do it often enough to be any good at it. He put the needle through the vein and infused the drug into my arm. Over the next few days, gravity pulled the stuff to my wrist and a progressive deterioration has been going on ever since. To this day, my wrist and thumb are becoming weaker and painful. But this doctor also referred me to a specialist. He said, "I see one or two myeloma patients a year. I want you to see someone who sees twenty to thirty a day." And the specialist to whom he referred me was Dr. James Berenson.

"Dr. B" tested the hardness of my bones. Mine were super hard. I don't know if it's genetics or being an athlete (I played for the Los Angeles Lakers with Wilt, West, and Baylor in the '68-'69 season). So, I am one of the few myeloma patients who doesn't take Zometa. My thoughts about my Santa Barbara oncologist are bittersweet. I stopped seeing him because he messed up my wrist but he put me in touch with one of the leading researchers/specialists in the country. I'd like to sue the Santa Barbara doc but I owe him. He got me to my myeloma guru.

Anyone with a unique disorder ought to see a specialist. At least get a second opinion. I used to drive from Santa Barbara to West Hollywood weekly. Now it's every other week. But it's so worth it. I would be really messed up by now if I hadn't been in the care of someone who knows what he is doing.

The next step was a bone marrow biopsy. Dr. B went into his version of the guy interrogating Kiefer Sutherland's Jack Bauer from the TV series *24*. He pulled out a drill (it's a Black and Decker clad in white), rolled me over, and bored a core out of my hip. I said, "I won't sign the papers or admit to anything. Jack Bauer is tough." Doc didn't get the joke but his attending nurse did and she started laughing. He said (while he was drilling), "Man, you've got thick, hard bones! Super dense. I've got to press harder." Then he switched gears and asked, "So, how do you think Kobe will do this year?" He wants to talk hoops while he is drilling. I inwardly smiled, then writhed and held back a scream as he pressed harder. Jack couldn't have done it any better.

A year later I didn't want to do it a second time, let alone a third a year after that. I was whining and moaning about having to have it done again and Dr. B said, "Ten years ago myeloma patients didn't live long enough to have more than one. This is your third." What could I say to that? So, he pulled out a drill and literally bored another hole in my hip. You have to have one each time you enter a new clinical trial.

Full-body X-rays showed no sign of bone lesions (myeloma tumors bore holes in your bones.) We had caught my disease early, it wasn't the aggressive kind, and I had hard bones. Although I didn't know it at the time, things could have been much worse.

My first drug treatment worked for six months but gave me neuropathy. Being an old athlete I was raised on "no pain, no gain." So, I made the mistake of not telling Dr. B about the progressing problem with my feet and legs until the condition was irreversible. I regret that a lot. I can still drive but walking is uncomfortable so I don't do it enough. Plus, I have serious balance issues.

When the first protocol began to fail it put me in a fetal position moaning. I had serious fatigue and felt awful most of the time.

The second protocol I was put on was on a clinical trial. It worked for five months but it too failed me. Understand that I didn't fail it. It failed me. It was at this time I wrote the following bit of nonsense:

(Warning: the following report contains multiple references to bodily functions and parts that tend to only be interesting to those who still think like junior-highers. Adults who continue to read do so at their own risk.)

I'm finding my combination of heart issues, cancer cures, and chemo have produced a plethora of naughty little nuisances that nag at me. I'll review a few.

It nags at me when I try to pee, while I pee, and when I am wrong about being finished peeing and then pee some more in my pants. Once a month I have to collect twenty-four hours' worth and keep it in the fridge. It's cause to pause before blindly reaching for the ginger ale.

It nags at me when I can't poop and when I can't stop pooping. Unlike Goldilocks and her porridge, I never get it just right anymore.

My nose is a nagging nuisance. How can it incessantly run and be plugged at the same time? I have to constantly blow, pick, swab, soothe, and assault it with a wide variety of sprays and salves. Having a naughty nose has raised an interesting question. When determining one's outlook on life, will having half a snoot full ever replace the age-old question "is the glass half empty or half full?"

Needles are a nuisance. Some shoot, some drip, but way too many are used way too often to take out way too much. I am what the angels disguised as nurses call "a tough stick." They tend to do a lot of fishing. That's what it's called when they come up dry and keep poking around. If I ever get pulled over for speeding the cop will take one look at my arms and automatically search my car for drugs.

All of my orifices are nuisances because they all have issues. Some itch, some burn, some have a rash, but most of them have either dried up or leak. "Red-eye" no longer conjures up thoughts of a late-night flight from Maui.

My largest organ nags me constantly. Every square inch of my skin itches like crazy. I need a device like a cone a vet puts on a dog to keep it from chewing on itself. I'm puzzled. How can I itch all over, feel tingly in some places, not feel anything in others, yet feel everything when it touches my skin? It hurts when I rub it but itches if I don't scratch. Go figure. My skin is bipolar.

I'm tired of being tired. Going for a walk with my wife is great but sitting on the curb while she gets the car because I can't get back up a little hill is a bit of a bother.

Balance is a nuisance. Hold it! That's not true. Not having much balance is the problem. I can't close my eyes to wash my hair in the shower without falling over backward.

My back hurts, my knees ache, and the things that should swell up don't, while the things that shouldn't do. It's a nuisance to hear my heart monitor beep on the hour, but I guess it would be worse if it didn't.

It's a nuisance to be quarantined. I'm susceptible to infections and my blood won't clot so I don't go to church or Bible studies. I don't do handshakes, groups, kids, planes, trains, or adults with sniffles. No eating genetically modified foods or anything sprayed with pesticides either. It is a big nuisance for this fast-food carnivore to be organic.

Finally, it's a nuisance when I set off metal detectors with my growing number of metal body parts. Just before starting chemo I drove all the way to Delano to minister to a prisoner but the guards wouldn't let me in because the screener beeped and I didn't have a letter from a doctor. They wouldn't pat me down. Nope. They just sent me home. Who knew?

I'll end my nuisance recital now. There are more but I'm annoying myself thinking about them all at once and I'm sure I've become a nuisance to you too.

Two and a half years ago Dr. B put me on another clinical trial. This was my third protocol and it was rough at the start. I had a one percent chance of getting pneumonia and a one percent chance of getting blood clots. Well, I got pneumonia and three blood clots in my lungs, plus a lung infarct the first week. First, I went to the emergency room, then spent four days in intensive care, and almost died.

Even after that experience, Dr. Berenson said he wanted to lower my drug doses and keep me on the same protocol while adding a blood thinner. I thought he was crazy but after chatting about it I said, "You're the doctor."

A month later I was greeted with good news. Dr. Berenson really liked my pee. And my blood, too. Everyone was raving about how much my bad myeloma test numbers had improved. Not quite what they would call remission, but very, very close. "Your numbers dropped off a cliff," were his words.

I am pleased to say three months later my bad proteins were at zero and I've had no measurable myeloma for over 27 months. That doesn't mean I'm cured. I still have the genetic defect that produces bad proteins. But the drug cocktail is killing the bad cells making those proteins before those cells and proteins can harm me. Now all I have to do is learn to deal with the side effects. At some point the drugs will probably stop working and then we will have to try another protocol. The good news is that there are other protocols to try.

I once asked Dr. Berenson, "What's the longest you have kept someone alive?" He replied eagerly, "I've kept my lawyer alive for twenty years!" I said, "Why?"

It took him a moment to realize I'd just made a lawyer joke. Then he laughed and said, "I can hardly wait to tell him."

I am now a "Cancer Coach" at my church. I help people get through the initial fear, shock, and anger of their encounter with the C-word. I'm finding an illustration of a dog helps the process.

Have you ever noticed that dogs don't spend any time in the past thinking about loss or regret? I have never seen a dog think about getting into the trash yesterday. That is a lesson for us. When I think about the past, I can't help but think about dumb things I've done and what cancer has taken from me. That kind of thinking is depressing and depression feeds my cancer. So, I try not to go there anymore.

Dogs don't seem to have any concern about the future either. I don't think I've ever seen a dog worry about tomorrow. That is another lesson for us. When I worry about what's going to happen to Mary when I'm gone or when I get concerned about the probability of being on morphine at the end, I start stressing out. But stress feeds my cancer. So, I try not to go there anymore either.

No, I want to think like a dog. I don't want to dwell in the past. And I don't want to wander into the future. I want to stay in the here and now and go for walks with my master.

What happens to a dog when his master says, "Do you want to go for a walk?" The dog gets uncontrollably excited. His rear end starts moving, his tail starts wagging, his feet start jumping, and the dog can hardly wait to go for a walk with his master.

That's me these days. I don't want to get trapped in the loss and regret of the past. And I try not to get caught in the anxiety of an unknown future. I want to take each day as it comes and wait for my Master to take me for a walk. And I have to tell you it is amazing how divine the encounters of the day become when the Master is walking the dog.

Everyone tells me I look good and don't appear to be sick. Actually, I'm not sure how to take that. It's a bit like saying, "Your face looks nice under all that makeup," "You don't sweat much for a fat guy," or, "Nice shirt, did you get it at the Goodwill?" Billy Crystal used to say, "Tis better to look good than feel good." So far Billy's been wrong, but I'll take what I can get. Neuropathy and fatigue are constant reminders that life isn't perfect. But I still have a remarkably high quality of life. I am productive and active in ministry. Life is full and good. At this point in time my "deadly disease" is really a "chronic disease." I was talking to my pulmonologist the other the other day and I asked, "Knowing my lung condition as you do, do you think a respiratory problem will kill me before my myeloma does?" He nodded affirmatively. It's a good thought to think myeloma probably won't kill me.

But there is a price to pay to stay alive. Part of that price is Dex. Dexamethasone, or "Dex" for short, is one of the drugs most myeloma patients have to take. It makes the other two drugs I have to take work better. But it messes with me.

The first time I took it the nurse told me I would start experiencing fatigue and nausea for a day or two, be sleepless, and have my period. Yes, you read it right. She said "my period"! That's as close as the nurse could get to explaining what was going to happen as a probable side effect. She said, "Was your wife ever irritable during her period?"

I figured this was a set up so I said, "Not my precious Mary." But some of my friends have mentioned it about their wives. The smile in the corner of my mouth gave me away and she said, "That's you for a short while."

Over the years, I have taken Dex and it has given me cataracts. I've already replaced my lenses once. It also eats muscle (my "guns" have become buggy whips), makes me retain water, causes a ravenous appetite, makes me gain weight, and gives me the male PMS symptoms the nurse talked about. I'm sleepless the day I take it and have an awful headache, I'm extremely irritable, have a very red face, experience hot flashes, have night sweats, and get an intense desire to watch the House and Garden Channel. I'm super hormonal and cry at the drop of a hat.

I was reading about a guy who gets so irritable his family calls him Tyrannosaurus Dex. And just this morning a neighbor and friend says she knows a guy who has myeloma and takes Dex on Fridays. His wife always leaves for the weekend.

So far, I'm doing okay with the irritability factor, or so says my dear wife. But I do watch a lot of "chick" shows on treatment days. Please, someone do an intervention if I start talking about having a sex change.

Taking strange drugs and experiencing strange feelings are only a part of the myeloma experience. You'll also have to participate in some very strange practices.

Myeloma patients have to collect their urine for twenty-four hours each month and bring it into the office. That reminds me of the man in the Alzheimer's wing of the long-term care home who was complaining about the bathroom light coming on when he goes in to pee a couple of times in the middle of each night. The maintenance man was baffled. So was the administrator. They both knew there is no automatic light in the bathroom. It stumped everyone until the cleaning lady opened the refrigerator door and discovered where the old man had been "going." Actually, I experience the illuminating part of that story each month. I have to admit I'd never envisioned myself making my middle of the night deposit into a plastic container in the kitchen illuminated from the light in the refrigerator while overcoming the chill of the escaping air. The absurdity of it all makes me laugh every time.

Last week I took in my monthly "24-hour collection." When you are 6'8", weigh 250 pounds, and have been ordered to hydrate, that's PC speak for a gallon of pee. My collection is under a strict protocol. It must be kept refrigerated, cooled in a picnic cooler when traveling, strapped in the seat for safety (the idea of that stuff flying freely in the car during a collision is a disturbing thought), and handed off to the lab tech. She always receives it with a smile and a warm greeting, but a pointing finger that says, "No, please don't set it on the table. Set it on the floor over there."

I broke protocol with the last collection. A breakfast meeting at IHOP with a dear friend went longer than I'd planned. When I stood up I knew I couldn't make it home in time. So, when we paid the bill I asked for a paper cup with a plastic lid.

"Would you like a straw?" the cashier asked?

"No thank you," I replied, and I could hardly keep from laughing as I dashed to the men's room.

As I exited, my friend walked in. I had my cup and I was on my way home to refrigerate its contents. My friend shook his head and started laughing. I did too. The cup was a spontaneous response to the need at hand. I hadn't planned for it. But it was fun.

Here is another fun thought. Short of something unforeseen, I'm planning to live another 10+ years even though the mortality charts give me 2 to 4. I'm currently with the right guy (Dr. Berenson) for my age and status. I'm not a candidate for the super aggressive treatment approach and wouldn't do it if I could. My guy thinks "less is best" and he has the stats to prove it. It fits me. If there is a study that will be better for me, Dr. B has the connections to get me in. There has also been talk of having a cure in the next five years. So, I'm a good candidate for that when it's ready. I'll stay close to my doctor.

Dr. Berenson is working on a cure and has actually cured laboratory mice. A friend asked, "How many mice has he cured?" I thought about that and responded with, "If it's a double-blind study, since there are three blind mice, at least six."

While I'm waiting for the cure I want to focus on being thankful for what I have, not what I've lost or don't have. And I want to remember great blessings come out of adversity. But it is not easy to think that way when there is so much loss.

Our daughter took a screen shot of Mary and me during a recent Skype session. Mary looks great. I have a fat puffy face and squinty, beady eyes. Steroids cause water retention and puffiness. So, I'm getting soggy and squinty. It's all part of continued, progressive, and unrelenting loss.

When you first hear the news that you have cancer you have to deal with shock, anger, and fear. But after you have had it for a while, you have to deal with loss. If you focus on how you have diminished, you won't do very well. It's important to focus on what you still have and what you still can do.

The Apostle Paul had an eye problem that God chose not to fix, even after repeated prayers for healing. But God used Paul in spite of his affliction. It doesn't look like God is going to heal me of my cancer, fatigue, or neuropathy, even after repeated prayers for healing. But like Paul, God is using me in spite of the afflictions. That's where the comparison ends as our impacts and responsibilities obviously differ. The great Apostle is an eagle of the faith. I'm an old buzzard. But words do not allow me to tell you how good it feels to be used by God to accomplish His will. Well, maybe I can. I can honestly say that the current opportunities to minister have made having cancer worth having. And that's a mouthful.

C. S. Lewis observes that "God whispers to us in our pleasures, speaks in our conscience, but shouts in our pains." Billy Graham said, "Comfort and prosperity have never enriched the world as adversity has done. Out of pain and problems have come the sweetest songs, the most poignant poems, the most gripping stories. Out of suffering and tears have come the greatest spirits and the most blessed lives."

Suffering often shifts our thinking from our immediate circumstances so we can listen to God concerning His work in our lives. Life as usual is replaced by a spiritual schoolroom. That's certainly been true in this stage of my life.

I think we go through what we go through to help other people get through what we went through." Those to whom God does not grant deliverance must learn to endure so that they can become ministers to those who are suffering from their affliction. Do you have a problem? Get ready to minister to someone who has your problem. That's probably why you have it.

Having ongoing treatments for an incurable cancer is like driving a convertible behind a truck carrying a couple of port-a-potties that are too high to get under the bridge ahead. You just never know what is going to get dumped on you next. I don't know what's coming next, but God does. He won't be surprised. And He promises it won't be more than I can bear. He also promises He will make something good out of it. So far so good on both counts.

I Have WHAT???

By John F. -- MULTIPLE MYELOMA?!!

Age: 40s

Publicist

Around June of 2009, I took a fall while hiking and believed that I fractured my rib cage. This seemed to take an awfully long time to heal, and then I had another fall around December of that year, resulting in agonizing pain in the upper back. So there was all this pain, but there were also falls that I could point to as the causes—I never suspected cancer. But still, the pain was getting worse and worse. Finally a chiropractor sent me for an MRI, which revealed multiple compression fractures in my thoracic spine. OK, now what? I saw many health care practitioners, but everyone missed what was really going on at that time. One thing I know for sure: excessive ongoing pain is not normal! Listen to your body; it always tells you what's going on. Always investigate and tell your physician about acute pain. If you feel something is wrong, insist on an MRI and blood work!

In February of 2010 (at the age of 43), I was feeling just really lousy overall. The pain was terrible, and now a general malaise had set in. I knew I needed to get to a hospital. My dear friends Denise and Nestor took me to the hospital. It's hard for me to even talk about this now, but the truth is I was in a near-death situation. At first, they wanted to send me home, as I didn't really look too sick. But blood tests, at the insistence of my friends, revealed otherwise. I was promptly admitted. Multiple myeloma, a blood cancer I had never even heard of, was the suspected and later confirmed diagnosis.

Myeloma left unchecked can grow really fast. Mine was of the lambda light chain variety, and this number was pushing 9,000 in the blood. (For those who don't know, the normal range is 5.71 to 26.3.) My blood counts were very low as well, and they asked me repeatedly to accept a transfusion, which I didn't want to do, but I finally relented.

Immediately following the transfusion, things went from bad to worse (coincidence?). All of my vital systems were failing, including my blood counts, kidneys, lungs, and heart. I had a black-out. Sepsis and pneumonia had set in, to compound the situation, and I believe I was in an induced coma. My plasma cells made up 90% of the bone marrow (normal is less than 1%). Chemotherapy was administered to me while I was in septic shock. This is risky business, but it did help. Finally I regained consciousness in the most miserable human condition you could possibly imagine. A slit had been cut in my throat to make way for an artificial breathing ventilator. I could not speak at all, of course, and was being "suctioned" all the time, a most unpleasant procedure to get rid of excess phlegm. What the hell was happening? I just lay there helpless, with no control over anything that went into or out of my body. I tried to tear everything out, but was restrained. I never knew this at the time but my family was told repeatedly that I probably wasn't going to make it. They put my chances of surviving the hospitalization at only 5%. "He's incompatible with life," they said. My family never allowed such negative prognostications to be spoken in my presence, thankfully.

As you can see, my immersion into the world of multiple myeloma was not a gentle or gradual one. There was no MGUS or smoldering myeloma grace period for me.

Luckily, my family and a few (very few) dedicated physicians, including James Berenson MD, didn't give up on me, and realized my life potential, in spite of the daunting odds. I had heard the name "Dr. Berenson" a lot while I was hospitalized. He is a world-esteemed myeloma expert physician, and I was told he had been to see me, and was consulting on my case. My sister Megan was in frequent mobile phone communication with Dr. Berenson. She informed me that after running in a local marathon one day, he just kept on going right up into my hospital room at Cedars to pay me a visit. I believe I was in a coma at the time, and don't actually remember the visit. Megan was astounded by the access level she had with Dr. Berenson, which was so greatly appreciated by her in those dark moments, when it was all so new and scary. Wherever Dr. Berenson was in the world, be it giving a keynote address at a medical conference in Istanbul or Vienna, he'd always take her call, or agree to speak at another mutually agreed upon time. What a comfort this was to my family, and a real act of dedication on the part of Dr. Berenson to his patients. Actually, all of Dr. Berenson's patients have his mobile phone number, something pretty much unheard of with other doctors.

My family was there in physical presence and also prayer. They had mobilized a vast network of prayers, and I felt this like a warm ocean blanket washing over me. That intensely healing spiritual energy, combined with the treatment with a custom-made combination of three drugs—Doxil, dexamethasone, and Velcade—that Dr. Berenson had developed, started to turn things around. My immune system, so under assault, kicked in, and I slowly started to improve. There were many mystical experiences that happened to me in the hospital, some you'd never believe.

I lay in that bed for months just staring. I was too weak and didn't care much about watching TV. Occasionally, I would scribble notes to my family or the medical staff. I desperately wanted to get out of there. I wanted the trach tube removed from my throat. But change and improvement came, slowly. After the "fade to black" period, I began to believe that I would, in fact, recover and get out of there. That was my intention, and psycho-spiritual power of intention was about the only tool at my disposal at that time.

I was also truly blessed with another angel physician, an infectious diseases specialist. Right from the beginning, the doctor took a strong interest in my case and was a fierce advocate for my well-being. I instinctively trusted the doctor, something I cannot say about many others. My doctors and Dr. Berenson were never afraid to buck the other doctors or the administration, in order to advocate on my behalf and secure the very best avenues for my care. I shudder to think what could have happened if I didn't have their guidance and navigation through the sometimes disjointed and illogical world of being a seriously ill patient in a major hospital. There was a doctor that had the guiding hand that directed me safely and smoothly throughout the ordeals of the hospital and to that happy day when I was finally able to return home. Oh, it was a long and protracted process, but I made it. I went from two different rooms in ICU, to the respiratory floor, to the 7th Floor Rehab, and then finally out the door (hopefully never to return!).

Hospitalization survival tips: Make sure your family visits frequently, because they will care more about you than others do; drink lots of water; get up and move around whenever possible; get outside in the sunlight every chance you possibly can; request essential oils and massages to feel connected to nature; listen to soothing music or watch comedy shows on TV (never the news!); and don't let them feed you cancer-fueling foods like breads, pastas, sugars, Ensure, etc.! (Even if you are new to this world, try to find out about anti-cancer foods, and don't think they'll serve you any, even in a cancer ward, if you don't request them. It's not that they don't care; they're just not educated about the importance of nutrition. It's up to you and those who love you to advocate on your behalf. Healthy food and water are essential.) And a final tip: Protect your right to sleep at night. Do not allow unnecessary nocturnal intrusions, because the body heals itself during sleep.

So I finally got out of the darkest period of my life and was ready to get back into the arena of reality. My first goal was get off the astonishing amount of prescription drugs that all the various specialists in the hospital had me on—yes, there was a "specialist" assigned to micromanage every system of my body. I've never been a fan of pharmaceutical industry drugs, and the fact that I was taking at least 15 different drugs greatly disturbed me. I weaned myself off this pharmacopeia, according to agreed plans with each prescribing physician.

Also around this time, my sister encouraged me to connect with Dr. Berenson. I called him on his mobile phone and expressed gratitude for everything that he had done for me during my hospitalization, and especially for all the kindnesses he extended to my family. Although I don't like drugs, I was in a desperate life-and-death situation, and the treatments prescribed by Dr. Berenson and other doctors really turned things around for me. This was the custom combination of Doxil, Velcade, and dexamethasone that had first been tried in the laboratory at the Institute for Myeloma & Bone Cancer Research (IMBCR) that Dr. Berenson runs, and was later successful in clinical trials under his direction. Every myeloma marker test in the hospital taken during this therapy had shown dramatic improvements and that I was responding! I began to realize I would, in fact, walk out the door of that place eventually—though this was hard to believe at times, especially with all the "code blues" going on, and the hugely uncomfortable feeling of seeing body bags taken out of rooms all around me.

I was grateful and lucky just to be alive. I wanted to use my PR skills to create a fundraiser for IMBCR. Dr. Berenson invited me over for a tour of his well-appointed offices on the Sunset strip, and also of the impressive IMBCR research laboratory. We then had lunch with Geoffrey Gee, IMBCR's Executive Director, to discuss the project. Dr. Berenson referred me to his wife Debra, whom I met not long after to hatch the plan. Debra is a very charming, fun-loving lady, an actress and a pianist, and we got along great. We decided on a Fall Art Benefit at the Andrew Weiss Gallery in Beverly Hills, and set out to make it happen.

Around this time, I was also referred to a brilliant naturopath named Dr. Bernardo. His life's work was exploring the missing links between conventional and alternative medicine. He used to say, "Cancer is not a death sentence, but it is a major inconvenience." Dr. Bernardo had been helping people reverse cancer for over 60 years. Immediately I went on Dr. Bernardo's protocol, which was a very strict alkalizing diet, with juicing, detoxing, and supplements. I reversed the acidosis that probably caused the cancer in the first place, and was amazed at how fast my lambda light chain levels dropped! (I was still in the range of 500 to 900 in the months since leaving the hospital before I went on Dr. Bernardo's plan. The first test after the plan showed it was below 100!) I was still receiving chemotherapy at this point; however, it became clear to me that an integrative approach was the only way to go. Nutrition is of *paramount* importance to the cancer patient. Everything we eat or drink either feeds disease, or prevents and reverses it. When one stops consuming junk, it's amazing how good you can look and feel.

So, our Fall Art Benefit at the Andrew Weiss Gallery for IMBCR was a great success. The show featured rare photos of Marilyn Monroe by her last living photographer, the estimable Bill Caroll, as well as a 20th Century Masters' collection featuring original works by Picasso, Miro, and Dali. About 70 people showed up, drank wine, nibbled on hors d'oeuvres, socialized, and bid on artwork. I particularly enjoyed working with the IMBCR staff on this, and it was also my first real opportunity to meet other myeloma patients.

By February 2011, I felt well enough to stop all chemotherapy. Continuing with my naturopathic plan, my lambda light chain remained very low—sometimes even as low as 35—for an entire year. A bone marrow biopsy in September 2011 showed extremely good results—plasma cells in the bone marrow were only in the single digits, maybe 4% or 5%. This was a glorious time, and proof that we as patients have a great deal to influence over how well we can do.

They say myeloma always comes back—something I never wanted to believe. But by January 2012, my lambda light chain levels shot up to 605. This was very surprising to me, as I was continuing my naturopathic protocol, maintaining alkalinity. I have a great knowledge of proper eating to stay alkaline, and had studied Ayurveda for the year prior, as well, incorporating healing Ayurveda teas and herbs into my regimen. Maybe it was some sort of psychological stress in December? Something appeared to have assaulted my immune system.

In April 2012, I decided to see if extreme whole-body hyperthermia could be an effective treatment for me. Myeloma can be hard to treat, harder than solid tumor situations, but whole-body hyperthermia made some degree of sense to me. I chose Germany over Tijuana, feeling that the environment there would be more conducive to my healing. After reviewing many clinics, I settled on the idyllically situated Dr. Herzog clinic in Bad Salzhausen, Germany. On arrival, my blood work looked great, and an ultrasound showed no issues in any organs. The problem was in the bones, and X-rays showed holes in my bones and osteoporosis. My walking had become difficult, and I had developed a pronounced limp.

The protocol in Germany involved complementary treatments like infusions with high doses of antioxidants and vitamins, infusions with homeopathic medications for detoxification, immunomodulation with xenogeneic peptides, magnetic field therapy, ozone therapy, oxygen therapy, and physiotherapy. And, of course, one treatment of extreme whole-body hyperthermia, where my body was heated to 107 degrees for an hour, with a simultaneous administration of a chemotherapeutic drug called bendamustine and the steroid prednisone. I woke up feeling amazingly well after this experience, and for the next several days—had no pain whatsoever and was actually walking perfectly normal.

However, after the first few days, I was limping again and the big blood test a week or so later revealed an alarming spike in the lambda light chain number. The doctor thought the elevation could be a result of cellular destruction. I wasn't sure—but did feel I was in some kind of healing crisis. Sometimes we get worse before we get better. The important thing is not to freak out, as attitude plays an enormous role in healing. Although I would have liked to have seen a dramatic improvement (as I witnessed many people there experiencing), I don't regret my experience in Germany and feel its value was more subtle.

Also while there, I was sent to Heidelberg to have a consult regarding a stem cell transplant. "The only known cures from myeloma have been as a result of stem cell transplants," I was told. I realize Dr. Berenson does not advocate transplants—but has not totally ruled it out. I was hoping to discover some new insights there, in what is regarded as one of the most cutting-edge transplant centers in the world. Ultimately I didn't learn anything I didn't already know—and the experience made me realize and appreciate the fact that I already have the best myeloma doctors and alternative healers in the world, right here in Los Angeles.

Back in LA, my lambda light chain continued its upward spiral. I resumed Velcade, and there was a dramatic improvement. Limping is almost gone now. Sometimes we have to do what we have to do. But also of enormous value was the implementation of: Chinese medicine, qi gong, Ayurveda, energy medicine, and complementary infusions of vitamin C, alpha-lipoic acid, and Traumeel. It's all about being open to whatever works. Integration is the best policy.

I believe multiple myeloma will be officially cured. It doesn't help anyone to believe in the "incurability" of any health condition, as our beliefs become our reality. Scurvy was very simply cured by vitamin C. Jonas Salk, after his wife developed polio, locked himself in a lab for six months and unlocked the riddle of the disease. The cure for myeloma already exists; it just needs to be discovered. IMBCR's *Cure Myeloma Project* has a great shot at being that discoverer, hopefully very soon!

I Have WHAT???

By John S. -- MULTIPLE MYELOMA?!!

Age: 70s

Retired Design Engineer

and Electronics Packaging Expert

What to start with? I guess my diagnosis, one of my sore points. Oh, not Dr. Berenson's diagnosis, I've no problem with that. It was accurate, speedy, and broke me out of a dither and into an effective and lasting relationship with him.

It is all the non-diagnoses that previous doctors had made for at least three years (perhaps as many as five). I first started having pain in my hips way back in 1993. In hindsight, it is easy to see this as the precursor to what was my multiple myeloma. I had to give up bike-riding but thought I was just getting old. I was 53. However, I still remained vigorous and physically active until 1999.

On an early August day in 1999, I got up to prepare for work. I rose at five to prepare for my morning routine, which consisted of shaving, then walking a mile, followed by a few floor exercises. Then it was time for my shower, breakfast, and off to work. My wife was on a slightly later schedule so our paths did not cross. My job title was Specification Engineer, but I also supervised design and drafting for two of my company's five product lines. It was an interesting job that I liked.

This morning was different. As I bent over the sink, I felt an electric tingle go up my lower spine, followed by a bolt of searing pain. I stumbled back to bed and called in sick. I saw my family doctor later that day. He assumed what I did: that I had a pinched nerve or pulled muscle in my 59-year-old back. He prescribed rest, pain meds, and a muscle relaxant and sent me home.

This was the first overt symptom of my MM but I can't blame my GP for missing it. In addition to the ambiguous symptoms, I have another problem: I look a good bit younger than my true age. Even now, at age 71, I have a full head of brown hair with just enough grey to prove I don't dye it. My face was, then, quite smooth and unlined. So I didn't look old enough to be a candidate for multiple myeloma, a common bias among non-specialists. Also, this doctor had only seen one previous myeloma patient, and that was when he was in medical school, many years before.

After some weeks, my back did not improve so my GP sent me to an orthopedic specialist. I had seen the ortho guy before for some shoulder and hip pain (clues?), but cortisone shots fixed those. He sent me for some X-rays and I came back to hear the news. He surprised me by asking me if I had ever taken a jolt to my back that was big enough to cause a collapsed vertebra. I could not name a time more recently than 25 years ago. He told me he didn't think it had caused my pain, anyhow. He then sent me for physical therapy, which may have been the worst thing he could do.

What the orthopedist did not do was read me the rest of the diagnostic radiologist's comments. I saw them two years later when I was gathering records for spinal surgery. The radiologist reported, among other things: "…there is moderate to severe osteopenia in the spine, hips, chest, ribs, shoulders, and skull." Had I seen those words in October 1999, you can bet I would have tracked the cause down and discovered my myeloma a lot earlier. I was feeling good enough to go back to work in November 1999, but I had a lot of back pain and general malaise.

In July 2001 I was forced to take a medical retirement. Luckily my employer's retirement plan included medical insurance. So for the next three months I dedicated myself to finding out what was wrong. My insurance system was a three-level setup: three different co-pay levels for HMO, PPO, and Out-of-Network. So I was referred to a different orthopedist. He sent me to a Sports Medicine specialist.

This guy sent me for tests and told me the first round was inconclusive. He gave me a list of what it might be. This ranged, from bad to worse, from a thyroid imbalance to multiple myeloma. He sent me for more tests. While I was going through every test and scan I could imagine, I made a decision. I would approach it from the worst possibility. I felt it would be easier to back down from that than to start at the least significant disease.

So I went online and found the International Myeloma Foundation. I found their Listserv and joined it. In the meantime, the new doctor was starting me on alendronate, a pill that is a bone strengthener for osteoporosis. At one meeting, which my wife attended with me, he slipped and referred to "your multiple myeloma." I stared at him, and he finally admitted that I really did have myeloma. It was like he was trying to protect me from the knowledge.

This annoyed me, and I decided to exercise my right to a second opinion. I went on the IMF Listserv and asked, "Who are the best myeloma doctors in the LA Basin?" The most mentioned oncologists were Drs. Berenson and Durie, both at Cedars-Sinai Medical Center. Dr. Durie was a biggie at the IMF and was reportedly not taking any new patients. Dr. Berenson was the Director of the Cedars-Sinai Myeloma and Bone Cancer program at that time and was taking new patients. I reached over and got out my insurer's PPO book. Dr. Berenson was in there as was Cedars-Sinai, in general. Gee, that was an easy decision to make!

I called and made an appointment with Dr. Berenson, and a few days later I was at Cedars-Sinai. He examined me, drew a good amount of blood, took some X-rays, and said he was certain I had multiple myeloma, but he wouldn't know how bad it was until the tests came back. I made another appointment with him for a couple of days later.

At the second meeting, he told me I was in bad shape. He didn't pull any punches, for which I was grateful. Trying to act in ignorance is one thing I abhor. I don't remember if it was the first or second visit that he did the bone marrow biopsy, but it supported the diagnosis. I was in Durie-Salmon Stage IIIA with significant bone damage: 12 compression fractures of the spine and very high blood test numbers. Eleven of those fractures had occurred since 1999. And I had shrunk five inches in height. My kidneys were very healthy, though. Dr. Berenson brought in Dr. Vescio, who agreed with it all.

In deciding what to do, I was dithering. Cedars-Sinai is a 40-mile drive on SoCal freeways from my home in Anaheim. This had the potential to become a hardship. But Dr. Berenson said something shocking, which probably saved my life: "I have a clinical trial going that would be perfect for you. But you have to have been off of your bone medication [alendronate] for three months, and you don't have three months to spare." This shocked me out of my dithering and I decided to make the 40-mile drive and stick with Dr. Berenson. This decision probably saved my life. I doubt I would have lasted six months otherwise.

Oh, that clinical trial Dr. B. mentioned to me? It was for a drug called PS-341. Today that drug is known as bortezomib or Velcade.

At the second meeting, Dr. B. told me that I needed aggressive treatment immediately. With the PS-341 trial an unlikely possibility for me, he offered to quickly set me up for a stem cell transplant (SCT). He said he was moving away from recommending SCTs but he thought it was best for my case. Unfortunately, the drugs used as part of the transplant procedure made my viral hepatitis infection become reactivated and my myeloma became very out of control. I became seriously ill during this time but fortunately with the use of the drug Epivir, both my viral hepatitis and myeloma came under control.

However, my myeloma eventually progressed and I participated in a clinical trial that brought my disease back under control. Since then, I have been a patient on many clinical studies during the past decade that have helped me. I am glad to have had the privilege of being part of clinical trials that have led to many therapies that are used to treat myeloma patients all over the world today. I appreciate the fact that Dr. Berenson has been able to have many of the newest drugs being tested for myeloma available for his patients. I know that there are many more drugs being developed in his research laboratory and others that will lead to even more options for me and other patients in the next few years.

I Have WHAT???

By Joyce F. -- MULTIPLE MYELOMA?!!

(Wife of 59½ years)

In memory of

Leslie (Les) F., beloved husband, father,

grandfather, brother, uncle, cousin

Age: 80s

English Professor (Purdue)

Les lived eight years after being diagnosed with multiple myeloma, for which his family will always be grateful. We doubt that without Dr. Berenson's ministrations, he would have lived this long. Les wrote his obituary five years before he died, and in it he wrote that he "felt secure that his multiple myeloma was being treated expertly under the direction of Dr. James Berenson in Los Angeles." He never wavered in that assessment.

This essay is written from the perspective of a wife, primary caregiver, case manager, data manager, fighter, cook of nutritious and organic foods, chauffeur, and bandager of wounds, as Les is, unfortunately, not able to write his own views. I will not focus on the specific treatments and medications and on the complications of other serious medical problems that Les had, but on the difficult tasks of coordinating Les' treatment from 1,800 miles away from Los Angeles with general oncologists in Indiana, where we lived, who were not myeloma specialists, and with other local medical specialists—nephrologists, gastroenterologists, cardiologists, neurosurgeons, dermatologists, speech therapists, edema specialists, etc.

The Beginning

In 2004, Les' health began deteriorating. However, it took many months before the diagnosis of multiple myeloma was made by a local oncologist, Dr. J, who was extremely uncomfortable in confirming this upsetting news. In a rush of words, he told me to read about it on the internet and by studying the pamphlets available in the clinic. He said his nurse would schedule an appointment at Indiana University (IU) Cancer Center with a myeloma specialist, and then he rushed out of the room. We were left numb and in a state of shock. His nurse came in and said she would contact IU and call us. The local oncologist would not begin any treatment until Les had been seen at IU. We went home, sat in the living room and cried, fearful of the unknown and sensing that our lives would never be the same.

As Les' kidney function was rapidly deteriorating week after week, Les had been seeing a nephrologist (i.e., kidney doctor) regularly, but she was reluctant to start any treatment until the myeloma was being treated. Her sole function, it seemed to me, was to schedule tests and discuss the results. We felt as if Les was a ping pong ball, being hit back and forth by the oncologist and the nephrologist, with neither willing to act rapidly and pro-actively nor neither one exhibiting any urgency.

After two weeks we still had not heard from the myeloma group at IU Cancer Center. I checked on this and discovered that the local oncologist's nurse had forgotten to contact IU, so I called the myeloma specialist's office directly and found out that he was on a long vacation and couldn't see Les for at least three weeks. I hung up, frustrated and angry but trying not to show my feelings and alarm to Les. Our children, Jeff and Lynda, were extremely concerned, and it was decided that we would have to seek treatment outside of our local area, West Lafayette and Indianapolis, Indiana. Jeff lives in Los Angeles and Lynda in New York, and so I found myself trying to negotiate on which coast we would seek a myeloma specialist. I rejected New York because of the difficulty for us of traveling in Manhattan to one of the cancer hospitals. In addition, neither Les nor I particularly liked the idea of getting treatment in an impersonal hospital setting.

I scoured the internet for days, reading articles and abstracts, and I kept finding articles by Dr. Berenson. I read about his approach to his patients and something clicked. I felt as if he would be a great fit for Les, who did not particularly like doctors in general and was very put off by the lack of people skills and compassion in the specialists that he had already seen. Jeff was also reading up on myeloma on the internet and coincidentally had also discovered Dr. Berenson. As luck would have it, Dr. Berenson had recently opened an office only blocks away from where Jeff and his family lived, and Dr. B. also had an affiliation with Cedars-Sinai Hospital, one of whose board members Jeff was acquainted with.

We concurred that Dr. B. would be the perfect match for Les, without any hesitation Jeff called the board member, explained the situation, and asked his advice on the best way to get Dr. B. to accept his father as a patient. Within 10 minutes, Dr. B. called Jeff and told him that it was *imperative* that Les begin treatment immediately to save his kidneys. He asked that I have all his medical records sent to him overnight and told Jeff that Les should fly to LA to see him the following week. As I recall, Dr. B. had a few choice words about the doctors who had sat on their hands for months! I remember talking to Dr. B. that same day and filling him in on the test results, and I recall how encouraged I was about his sense of urgency and his concern for his new patient.

There was an immediate complication associated with Les' trip to LA. I would not be able to accompany him, as I was having a procedure done by an interventional radiologist on my left hip to ease considerable pain until I could undergo hip replacement surgery. I had decided to postpone any thoughts of surgery until Les' course of treatment was underway. My orthopedic surgeon reluctantly agreed to use various techniques to control the pain so I could function and help Les until that time. The procedure was to be done in the hospital outpatient facility and had been scheduled weeks before. If I cancelled, I might have had to wait several weeks before it could be re-scheduled. Therefore, it was decided that Jeff would accompany his father to Dr. B. and would have to take good notes for me. That was the first and last time that I did not go with Les to any medical appointment.

Before Les' first appointment with Dr. B., we had already changed oncologists. A friend of ours, who also had multiple myeloma, had recently switched to the highly recommended Dr. R. Les found her more compassionate than Dr. J. and certainly more willing to take the time needed to explain and comfort the patient. What she lacked in experience she made up for in compassion and people skills and a willingness to work with Dr. B. Of course, she was in awe of Dr. B. and understood our need to work with a myeloma specialist. All the local oncologists worked with patients having the whole gamut of cancers and did not specialize.

When Les returned from LA with specific instructions for chemo treatment and various meds, Dr. R. became the primary local contact for ordering the infusions, assorted meds, and frequent tests, and monitoring his condition.

By this time, we had also changed nephrologists. Dr. A. was the total opposite of the previous nephrologist—proactive, thorough, and willing to cooperate with Dr. R. and Dr. Berenson. Les was comfortable with Dr. A. and they often shared their remembrances of Wayne State University, where Les received his BA and Dr. A completed his residency. There was a wonderful comfort level between Les and Dr. A. This was important as Les was able to open up and discuss his emotions and physical problems with Dr. A.

The difficult part was getting the lab results immediately sent to Dr. B. and me. The nurses and support staff of the doctors at the clinic were not used to a patient's caregiver expecting that all lab reports be faxed to another doctor and her. But I was persistent and we worked out an accommodation after a while. The lab results were faxed only to me, and then I faxed them to Dr. B. for his review. I know that I was a pest and I added an extra burden for these extremely busy nurses and office staff, but as I had taken on the role of "case manager" I felt I absolutely had to get the results to Dr. B. as soon as possible. I guess I was the pit bull, but the 1,800 miles between LA and West Lafayette, Indiana required timely coordination among all the physicians.

Les endured many "collateral" problems that wore him down physically and emotionally, making him feel helpless and afraid that he would lose control over his life. Les had taught at Purdue University for about 36 years and enjoyed the freedom to do what he wanted in retirement. He walked, rode his bike, read the entire *New*

York Times daily, read books that he had intended to read and re-read after he retired, watched movies, listened to classical music and opera, and relished his freedom to do whatever he loved to do, without the "distractions" of preparing lectures, grading papers, and attending those departmental meetings. That sense of freedom was seriously jeopardized when his life focused on treating the myeloma and his kidneys. As the years moved on and he had more courses of chemotherapy and maintenance treatment, and developed other challenging health problems, the deterioration that occurred in his quality of life and lifestyle caused him great anguish and vanquished his peace of mind.

During the first course of chemotherapy, he had sores in his mouth and for a few weeks had difficulty eating anything but soft foods and liquids. Then he could not taste his food and complained that I no longer seasoned it. He didn't want to eat out as he couldn't taste anything, he said. Les no longer enjoyed anything I cooked for him. Another problem arose during the second infusion: the needle for the Doxil came out of his arm and seriously burned the skin on his forearm. We were leaving the next day for LA and on the plane we were putting ice packs on his scarred arm. He was in pain for weeks. The day after our arrival Les had an appointment with
Dr. B. He was justifiably furious about the Doxil spill. He had many piercing adjectives, as you can imagine, for the infusion lab staff in our clinic that hadn't monitored Les properly. We all know that Dr. B. does not suffer fools or incompetents! Dr. B. made an immediate appointment with a local dermatologist to look at Les' burns that

same day. Another specialist for Les to see! He saw this as another unwelcome intrusion into his time to relax and visit with his family in LA.

The aggressive treatment prescribed by Dr. B. worked, as Les went into remission after three courses of treatment; however, what is indelicately called "chemo brain" persisted for many months. That side effect necessitated banning him from driving, as he could no longer reliably focus on stop signs and stoplights.

The myeloma had to be treated numerous times during the eight years following its diagnosis. And we changed oncologists frequently. Dr. R. moved on to a position in another clinic so that she could specialize in breast cancer. Les was then treated by Dr. K., who had a warm and compassionate demeanor and could draw Les out. He also was quite willing to work with Dr. B., and to administer what he humorously called "Dr. Berenson's cocktail." He didn't always understand why Dr. B created his own treatments but he followed them, nevertheless.

He was very sensitive to Les' successive problems and stayed on top of Les' treatment and side effects. Les had developed severe edema in his ankles, to the point that he could no longer walk out of the house wearing any of his shoes. Dr. K. referred him to edema specialists who bound his feet and saw him three times weekly for three weeks, until the swelling had totally disappeared. Of course, thereafter Les always wore heavy compression socks, which he hated, especially in the summer.

Les also developed severe back problems and leg pains. He was seen by Dr. C., a neurosurgeon, who had years before successfully operated on my spinal stenosis, and I wanted to have him operate on Les. Interestingly, Dr. C. saw on the X-rays what others, including an interventional radiologist, did not see. Not only did Les have a compression fracture but he also had a disc issue that was causing the leg pain and which could be repaired at the same time. The surgery was successful, but took an emotional toll.

While under Dr. K.'s care, as he was trying very conscientiously to determine the source of Les' shortness of breath, a lesion was detected in one lung. None of the tests revealed the exact location, size, or whether this was a cancerous growth on the lung. Considering Les' medical history, the oncologist, Les' internist, and the thoracic surgeon agreed that surgery was the best course of action. Les was extremely apprehensive and internalized his fears and concerns. It was almost impossible to get him to talk about what he was feeling and he was irritable most of the time leading up to the surgery. We arrived at the hospital early in the morning as Les was supposed to be the surgeon's first patient that day, but the surgeon had to perform an emergency procedure which delayed Les' surgery. Then that patient experienced some problems, which necessitated being returned to surgery. Les spent the entire day waiting and worrying. When he finally was taken into the surgical suite, the procedure was quite rapid. Luckily, there was no cancerous growth. It was a lesion from a bout of pneumonia that had occurred many years ago.

Les didn't arrive in the recovery room until after 7:00 p.m., and at that late hour he was the only patient in the entire large recovery area. As he began to come out of the anesthesia, he called for me and wanted to know whether he had another cancer.

I reassured him that everything was benign but he was reluctant to believe me. It was then that I realized how worried and afraid he had been of the outcome. The pain medication had him hallucinating and talking non-stop about all sorts of things from his past, and the hilarity of his reminiscences kept me and the recovery nurses laughing and joking with him. A lot of my tension and weariness lifted. I stayed with Les that night, but the pain medication (morphine drip, I think) kept him semi-awake all night, chattering constantly, and I got very little sleep. The floor nurses kept coming in as they were really amused by his anecdotes and descriptions of people and events. It was a surreal free association night. Too bad that Dr. Freud wasn't there. The next day our daughter arrived and she starting giggling at Les' hallucinations and chattering. She said laughingly, "Mom, Dad is high." I looked incredulous, but she insisted that he was on a morphine high!

The healing of the incision took quite some time and restricted his mobility somewhat. He was not too happy having me bathe and dress him. He felt he was losing control and that his body had become his enemy. He was fighting to retain his independence while knowing that he was becoming more physically dependent. That was difficult for this very proud and independent man and for me, his wife, to see. He never wanted to be a burden on anyone and he could not accept that he needed assistance in some personal areas of his life. But he also would not try to help himself become stronger by undertaking a regular exercise program, for instance, or walking outside.

After working with Les for about three years, Dr. K. decided to move to a small practice in a smaller town in western Canada so that he would have more time to spend with his family. This didn't leave us with many options, so we chose Dr. V. K., by default. The first visit with her made it very clear that Les would not be comfortable working with her. She was rather cold, standoffish, argumentative, and dismissive, and her ego seemed to be bruised when we told her that she would be taking directions from Dr. B. But events, fortunately and unfortunately, moved us into the hands of a remarkable oncologist who had only recently joined the clinic. I had heard of his reputation and wanted to switch to him when events unrelated to Les' myeloma overtook us.

Les had a stroke, which affected his language center very briefly but was devastating to Les emotionally. Two excellent specialists became frequent visitors to Les' hospital room—the neurologist, Dr. H. (whose wife is a good friend), and the oncologist Dr. H., who was the oncologist on call that weekend. This oncologist immediately hit it off with Les and me. His calm and compassionate manner reassured Les and we instantly decided that we would change oncologists. That decision proved to be fortuitous. As soon as he put his arm on my shoulder and said, "I will take good care of Les and make sure that he has proper attention to his condition," I put my trust in him.

Les had an office visit with Dr. H. a few days after he was discharged from the hospital, at which time I explained to him the role that Dr. B. played in Les' treatment. Right then he turned on the internet on his computer and began checking on Dr. B. He was amazed by Dr. B.'s professional reputation and wanted to know how we got a doctor of his reputation to accept a patient so far away! We explained the whole sequence of events and then I gave him Dr. B.'s cell phone number and suggested that he call him immediately.

He was even more amazed when I told him that Dr. B. gave all of his patients his cell phone number. Dr. H. has a very expressive face and as his eyebrows rose, you could see him processing that remarkable and unique feature of Dr. B.'s patient care. He kept asking whether I thought it was appropriate for him to call Dr. B. so early in the day. I assured him that the best way to coordinate care would be to introduce himself to Dr. B. on the phone. Dr. H. left the room and after five minutes he returned, beaming and full of pride. Apparently, he had made an instant connection with Dr. B., who had even suggested that they work together on a clinical trial. This was a tremendous coup for Dr. H., of course, and assured us that the transition to Dr. H.'s care would be effortless. (A few months later I found out that Dr. H. and Dr. A., Les' nephrologist, had graduated in the same medical school class and were friends, so they were able to coordinate regarding Les' treatment with no difficulty.)

Later that day I received either a phone call or an email from Dr. B. saying that he was glad we finally had an intelligent and competent oncologist to work with! He was never one to mince words or be "politically correct," which Les appreciated. Les found Dr. B.'s honesty, quick mind, and humor very refreshing. And Dr. B. liked talking to Les about literature and art. So they always were comfortable with each other.

The first night in the hospital—I detected Les had had a stroke about 8:00 a.m. on a Saturday morning of a holiday weekend—was interesting. I left the hospital about midnight, hoping to get a few hours' rest at home, after Les was stabilized and comfortable. When I returned about 6:00 a.m. the following day, the nurses were full of stories about Les' evening. He had hardly slept but they kept hearing voices in his room and went in to check on him. He was pronouncing the names of all his family members and then reciting famous speeches from Shakespeare's plays to work on his speech. He wanted to surprise me by showing that his speech had not been seriously impaired. His will to return to "normal" was remarkable.

He did have some speech problems but speech therapists started working with him immediately on Sunday morning. After his discharge from the hospital, a speech therapist came to the house twice weekly for a number of weeks to work with him. The problem arose when he was able to visit a speech therapist at the clinic. We went to a few appointments but it soon became obvious that he did not want to cooperate with that plan. He was weary of the time taken away from his reading for doctor visits and therapy sessions. So he went only so far and then balked. The speech therapist realized that he was unwilling to continue (he felt the exercises were juvenile); and, therefore, we compromised: he agreed to practice his speech exercises with me at home and to read aloud a few times a day. Over time his speech improved tremendously. He spoke a bit slower and sometimes he forgot a word or two, but unless someone had known him for many years past, no one would have surmised that he had had a stroke. However, it seemed to his family that his mental sharpness began deteriorating and that as new health issues arose in quick succession, he was physically declining. Whether this can be attributed to the stroke or other issues, we did not know.

Our children noted that, as a result of the stroke, Les had difficulty initiating a conversation. The therapist said it was quite common and Les admitted to it. More often than not, he responded to a discussion rather than started one. And it was much more difficult for him to process complex ideas and verbalize abstract or conceptual thoughts.

He suffered from many problems unrelated to his myeloma, including thyroid problems, dehydration, excessive bleeding from slight scratches and bruises, difficulty swallowing food, loss of appetite, falls, general weakness, shortness of breath, dizziness, difficulty with balance, and frequent stays in the hospital. As he became weaker, he became more sullen and unhappy. He had always been an intensely independent and private person. As he became more dependent on me or a home health aide to help him bathe and bandage his "wounds" every day, or to help him manage using his walker to get out of the house into the car for his multiple visits to the lab for tests and to the assorted doctors for medical appointments, he railed against his diminished quality of life. Everything that had given him so much pleasure in life was ebbing away. When he found it difficult to read and retain what he had read, I think his will to live gave out. He often said he had never imagined that he would have a lingering illness that would mar his retirement years. He wanted to leave on his own terms, but as his body became his enemy, it defeated his spirit.

Watching my beloved husband deteriorate and live in constant physical pain was the hardest thing I had ever lived through. I tried not to show Les my own weariness, fears, and heartbreak, but we had lived too many years together for him not to sense my emotions. He didn't want to discuss how I should handle all the books and personal papers in his study. I don't think he could ever face that those objects would no longer be in his study. To this day, a year after his death, I cannot face discarding any of the books and papers that defined his professional and personal life, as I fear that emptying his study will cancel his existence on earth. I know he is at peace now but I cannot forget how much he suffered. Les and I shared many interests and values, and a day does not go by that I don't think of him, especially when I read something interesting that we might have discussed, hear an aria that we both loved, or watch a movie that I know he would have enjoyed. I pick up a book and read his marginal comments, some of them addressed to me, and I sense what he was thinking as he read the book. I never met another person who had such a compelling dialog with the writer of each book that he was reading. The children and I always laughed that Les had to find a literary analog for anything he experienced in the "real" world. That was part of his charm. Multiple myeloma didn't change his unique way of thinking and living, but it did hasten his death.

"Pace, pace," my dear soul mate.

I Have WHAT???

By Karen S. -- MULTIPLE MYELOMA?!!

Age: 60s

Retired Special Education Teacher

For years my husband, Therman, and I had dreamed of selling our home and moving into a motorhome when we retired. In July of 1998 we started our adventure. Our motor home allowed us to travel around the United States, enjoying the sites of this wonderful country we live in.

We kept our boat, so we spent each summer at a lake near Eugene, Oregon. Our kids, their wives, and our nine grandchildren would join us at the lake. We played games, spent time on the boat waterskiing, wakeboarding, and playing on the tubes. The grandkids looked forward to their time at the lake with their cousins. We were living our dream.

In 2004 my white count was low, so my doctor referred me to a hematologist. I was shocked when I arrived at the clinic and the sign said hematology and oncology. I reasoned that they must share the clinic and that I wasn't seeing an oncologist. After reviewing my records, asking me many questions during an hour interview and examining me, he, the oncologist, could not see any reason for the low white count. He said he had another patient with a low white count and she was doing fine. He was intrigued by how active I was and loved the fact that I water-skied and had just learned to wakeboard. He felt that there wasn't anything seriously wrong. He ordered 26 blood tests and said that he didn't see a need for a bone morrow biopsy. I was excited until I received a call a couple days later telling me I needed that biopsy. My first reaction was to stop chasing this allusive "problem"' because I felt fine. But what if this test revealed a problem?

A few days after the test I had an appointment with the oncologist. I was nervous and it didn't help that he was running an hour late. I was somewhat relieved when he bounced into the room and the first thing he asked was, "Well, have you been wakeboarding?" I told him, "Yes, I have been on the wakeboard, but I am here to find out the results of my bone morrow biopsy." He realized that the nurse hadn't printed out the results so he left the room to get the information.

It felt like an eternity before he finally returned. The second time he entered the room he wasn't so happy. He was having a hard time coming up with words. He talked about why I was referred to him and blah, blah, blah. He finally said, "They have a name for what you have—multiple myeloma." I didn't know what multiple myeloma was but I was sure it wasn't good by the look on the doctor's face. Therman asked if it was cancer. After hearing the doctor say it was cancer I felt tears on my cheeks. I can't remember everything that was said but one of the things I heard was the doctor telling Therman that when he has seen myeloma patients they were in a world of hurt. I remember him telling us that there was no cure but there were lots of new treatments available. He ordered more blood tests and a bone survey to be done before we left the clinic. I was in shock. As I lay on that cold X-ray table while they took 13 X-rays, I was trying to make sense of the information I had just received.

Cancer—no cure—how much time do I have—will I live long enough to see my grandchildren grow up—will I have to have chemo—will my hair fall out—what was life going to be like now that I have cancer? What was Therman thinking? It just broke my heart to see the pain in his eyes. He held my hand as tight as we silently walked to the car. As I sat sobbing a gentle hand touched my shoulder. When I looked over at Therman there were tears in his eyes, too. We were in shock and just couldn't wrap our minds around a diagnosis of cancer. It was a long drive back to the lake.

The first thing I did was get on the computer. It wasn't long until I read about a treatment center that was bragging about keeping their myeloma patients alive for three years. Three years, I only had three years if I am lucky? I woke Therman up and told him what I had found. I said, "When you remarry, please protect our children's inheritance."

By the next morning, I was a basket case. I needed answers. I called my doctor's office but he was on vacation, and the nurse wasn't that familiar with myeloma so she was no help. I found a cancer counselor and she was wonderful. After helping me deal with a cancer diagnosis, she gave me information about the Leukemia & Lymphoma Society support group. I called the leader of the Portland group and she was so encouraging and supportive. She sent me a packet of information and asked if it would be okay to have their First Connection Person call me. Within an hour, I received a call from Julie. She was able to help me by sharing what she had experienced with myeloma. She gave me hope.

It was time to meet with the myeloma specialist for a second opinion. I remember telling her that I was there for one reason and one reason only—for her to tell me my doctor was wrong and that I didn't have myeloma. She had to deliver the bad news that my doctor was correct but that it was early and at this time I should not have treatment. NOT HAVE TREATMENT? I had cancer and she said that I shouldn't have treatment? That didn't make any sense to me. She spent an hour explaining myeloma to us and said that treatment at that time was unnecessary because the cancer wasn't causing any major problems and treatments had side effects. She also shared with us that there were new more effective treatments available when and if needed. A message of hope!

After frequent blood tests over the next year, it was obvious that I had what was called smoldering myeloma which meant that it was not active, it was like being in remission.

While in Portland we attended a support group. Dr. James Berenson was the guest speaker at one of the meetings. Therman and I were very impressed by what he had to say and it was the first time I heard a myeloma specialist recommend not having a transplant. He was so positive and talked about "quality of life." He also talked about using fewer drugs, which would not do harm, and how that approach would allow other treatments to be given later on when the current one failed to work. What he said made sense. We liked what we heard.

For the next 4½ years after being diagnosed with myeloma, I had blood and urine tests as well as bone surveys on a regular basis. The myeloma progressed at a slow rate.

On January 9, 2009 (my birthday), while getting ready for a hike in Big Bend National Park in Oregon, I injured my back. I was changing into my capris when I felt a snap in my back with pain shooting to my hip. I thought I had pulled a muscle. I didn't think it was a bone problem because I had a bone survey less than six months earlier. So I continued hiking. I managed the level ground fine but when it was time to scramble up and over the rocks, the pain increased and I became nauseated. I just thought I needed to rest. I tried to hike the next day and ran into the same problem. Crazy me, it turned out to be a compression fracture in my spine.

When I arrived at the clinic in Arizona, I had a CT/PET scan. There were two areas of concern, the compression fracture of T12 and a large lesion in my right hipbone. I knew it was time for therapy, but it felt like a punch in the stomach when the doctor said it was time to start treatment. I was afraid it would interfere with our travels. But I knew it was necessary. The first thing I did was start radiation on my hip.

I asked about being on a clinical trial but because my absolute neutrophil count was so low I could not qualify for any of the trials. The oncologist said that my treatment options were very limited because of my low counts. He recommended that I start a high dose of thalidomide along with dex. I told him that I wanted to think about it and would get back to him.

After talking it over with my husband, I agreed to try it even though I felt that the dose was too high. I will never forget that day. Tears were streaming down my face as I put that pill in my mouth. I realized that my life was now changing and I would be dealing with medicines, side effects, and doctor's appointments. After a week of this treatment, the side effects (severe fatigue, tingling in my feet and hands, tingling around my lips) were too much for me, so I left a message for the doctor that I didn't want to continue thalidomide. He said to stop taking it for a week and meet with him. We revisited the pros and cons of each of the drug options with him recommending that I stay with the thalidomide at a lower dose. I thanked him for the information and told him I would think about it.

Again after talking it over with Therman, I decided to give it another try at the lower dose. I was able to tolerate it but the side effects were still hard to manage. It seemed to work for the first couple of months but by the third round of treatment it was obvious that the drug had stopped working. When I went off of thalidomide, my myeloma test numbers went higher than they were before I started taking it.

Next, we decided that I would start Revlimid with dex when we arrived back in Oregon in June of 2009. What a pleasant surprise when I discovered that the side effects were very mild (leg cramps being the most bothersome one). I scheduled the kids' and grandkids' visits to the lake around my doctor's visits. No visitors on my dex crash days. My grandkids loved being with me on my two "high" dex days and wanted to stay up all night with me on those nights. I was thrilled that the summer wasn't disrupted by my treatment. In fact, I was able to water ski and wakeboard. I wasn't sure I would be able to after having a compression fracture just six months earlier. Therman tried to talk me out of it but after I reassured him that I would be careful, he gave in. Therman is needed because he is the boat captain (driver). I really enjoyed being back on the skis and the wakeboard—it made me feel normal.

By the end of the summer, the Revlimid treatment had brought my numbers down but had not put me into complete remission.

I had several discussions with my oncologist about a transplant. He wanted me to get one as soon as possible. I wasn't interested at that time. I felt that with the available drugs, the new ones soon to be available, and the information from Dr. Berenson, there might not be a need for a transplant. However, I was not ready to completely take the transplant option off the table, so decided to have my stem cells collected.

When I went off of Revlimid to prepare for collection, my cancer numbers went right back up. I had to go on to bring my numbers down before collection. This new drug posed a real challenge because of its side effects. I was on weekly infusions and was very sick for a few days after each treatment. I had problems with vomiting, diarrhea, and nausea.

I just couldn't imagine a good summer with our family with these weekly side effects. So, before heading to Oregon in June 2010, I discussed my concerns with my doctor and was able to reduce the dose of Velcade, and he added Cytoxan. I did so much better and my side effects were not so severe.

On January 2011, I was able to go from weekly treatments to every other week. I loved having more time between my visits to the clinic for treatments, which allowed us to do more traveling. It was a delicate balance between keeping the myeloma in check and maintaining quality of life. It was important to me to get this right.

By the end of the year, my cancer numbers were slowly creeping up. I was feeling fine when I thought I had an ear infection. We headed to the emergency room where they discovered spinal fluid coming out my ear. The CT scan showed that I had air in my brain. They transferred me to Tucson, Arizona where I had surgery to patch the holes. I ended up with an abscess in my brain. I was taken off of my cancer treatment for the month of December. After 12 days in the hospital I finally was able to go home, but had to be on daily IV antibiotics for 10 weeks.

In January 2012, I was back on weekly cancer treatments. I was having some real problems with side effects from the three heavy-duty antibiotics—or were some of them from the myeloma? My red count, white count, and platelets were low. My kidneys weren't functioning properly and my heart rate was very high. I was scared. I remember lying in bed wondering if I would survive. I felt horrible. After the first week in February, I was taken off of the antibiotics. The MRI done three weeks later showed that the abscess was gone. I was thrilled.

At the end of March, I had recovered enough to be able to fly to Oregon to visit our kids and grandkids. My kidney function was improving and I was back to walking 20 minutes per day.

In April, Therman and I flew to Williamsburg, Virginia. What a thrill it was to be traveling again and enjoying the history of our great country. A few days after returning and getting my treatment, we visited family in Texas. I was able to see all of my siblings and Therman's siblings along with his 92-year-old mother. Then, it was back to Arizona for my next treatment.

My cancer markers were bouncing up and down, with more ups than downs. The last couple of labs were up. I have to admit that I was scared. *Will the next drug combination work? If not, then what?* I still get those sweaty palms and feel a little uptight before each lab test.

At my last doctor's appointment, we made a plan to decrease the Velcade in order to add Revlimid and to stop the Cytoxan.

My oncologist is still pushing me to get a transplant, but I am refusing. When the pressure gets too great, I just listen to some of Dr. Berenson's interviews. He keeps me focused on the positive and helps support my decision not to have a transplant. He gives me such hope. I consulted with him a couple of years ago, attended some of his presentations, listened to all of his interviews on Patient Power, and I plan on meeting with him when I need more advice.

I feel that it is so important to have a strong support system. It is support that helps me deal with this crazy, unpredictable cancer. I belong to a support group in Arizona, one in Oregon, and a worldwide online support group. I also have a group of friends and family members I share my journey with. They send me encouraging e-mails and notes and share their trials with me.

My sons and daughters-in-law have been so supportive. They pitch in while at the lake, helping with meals and clean-up. They are there offering any help needed.

My grandkids are awesome. They have done things like: sign the promise to support the search for a cure in her Nana's honor when the Lance Armstrong team came to her school, donate blood, make and sell friendship bracelets to raise $25 for a cure, write a paper for one of their classes about myeloma, run five miles for their Nana and gave me the medal, attend a myeloma workshop with me and give a speech about how Nana inspires them, just to name a few. One day, the little one crawled into my lap, threw her arms around my neck and said, "Oh Nana, I wish you didn't have cancer." When I was having problems with side effects, my high school granddaughter offered to get me some "helpful substance." I just couldn't imagine asking her to do something illegal, but I love the thought that she cared enough to offer. I enjoy their love, support, encouragement, hugs, and kisses.

My number one supporter is Therman. He goes to all of my doctor appointments, helps me research information about myeloma, and is there for me on those rough days. He's my husband of 48 years, lover, travel companion, and best friend.

Getting support has really made a difference in my life.

We are still living our dream, but it is a dream with modifications. We take mini trips now as we enjoy the sites of Arizona while in the Southwest. We work our activities around my treatments. Last fall we wanted more travel time, so I made arrangements with an oncologist in Salt Lake City to get my Velcade treatment while traveling through there. We were able to spend a couple of weeks traveling up north including a week at Yellowstone before getting my treatment. After resting a couple of days, we had two more weeks to enjoy the canyon country. One of our hikes took us to a little known formation of rock art called "Five Faces." We met our friends there and did a little off-roading with them before heading to Arizona. There is life after a cancer diagnosis!

We still live in our motorhome, we still spend our summers at the lake with our family, and we still enjoy traveling. The dream is still alive, but now includes helping in finding a cure for multiple myeloma.

I Have WHAT???

By Linda R. -- MULTIPLIE MYELOMA?!!

Age: Late 50s

Retired Teacher

The quintessentially healthy 56-year-old…that was me. I was 3½ years into retirement after a rewarding teaching career, I traveled the world with my husband, we had two beautiful grandsons…it was the perfect life. But that pesky anemia…always there at every yearly physical. I didn't give it two seconds of thought, because my blood count had always been rather low. It didn't concern me at all. I felt great, and life was better than good.

In July of 2002, it was again time for my yearly checkup. For the past year, my primary care doctor had tried everything he could think of to get to the bottom of my anemia. There was no readily apparent cause, and no amount of iron was helping the situation. Such an insignificant thing to me, but it bothered him a lot. He finally told me he just didn't feel right about it and was referring me to a hematologist. So off I went to the "hem/onc" (that's medical speak for a hematologist/oncologist), still not at all concerned, because I felt absolutely fine. Several blood tests and a bone marrow aspiration later, I received the news. I had Stage 2 multiple myeloma. Me???? But I felt so good! How could I have an incurable cancer that I'd never even heard of? We began to do some research, and the news at the time was depressing. Yes, I was scared, but I decided right then and there that I wasn't going to be a part of "their" statistical pool. I declared to my new doctor that I was going to be his "star" patient, and asked him what did I need to do? He told me that an autologous stem cell transplant would be my best option. I trusted him completely. So I said, let's go!

Within two weeks of diagnosis, I was in the hospital receiving my first of three rounds of VAD chemotherapy, which was the gold standard at the time. This was a concoction of vincristine, Adriamycin, and oral dexamethasone. After three rounds my numbers were down sufficiently enough that I was deemed "ready to prepare for the transplant." My stem cells were collected, there was more chemo and drug therapy, and then in March of 2003 I received my own stem cells back after several heavy-duty hits of intravenous melphalan cleaned out my bone marrow. I spent 15 days in the hospital and came out feeling great. Even losing my hair wasn't as bad as advertised…more like an interesting adventure. Truthfully, when my hair grew back I found myself resenting it all the time with the hair dryer! Within six weeks, I was back on the risers singing with my beloved Sweet Adeline's Chorus, and that summer we took a memorable trip to Europe. I continued to receive monthly infusions of Zometa, and there was no sign of myeloma in my bone marrow. This glorious remission lasted for three years.

In January of 2006, my labs suggested there might be something amiss. Yes, indeed, "it" was back. We watched the steady climb of my IgA number for the next year and then in early 2007 it became apparent that we needed to do something. My transplant doctor suggested another transplant. I was now 61 years old and not at all sure that I wanted to put my body through that again, but if not that, then what? It was then that we decided to go see Dr. James Berenson.

It was a good decision. Even the phone call to make the first appointment made me feel that I would be in good hands, such is the caring, positive manner of his whole staff. And I was so right. Dr. Berenson's approach was much more conservative. Because of his extensive knowledge and research in the area of myeloma, he is able to suggest individualized therapies for his patients. He felt that the new drugs that had been approved would be just as, or more effective than, another transplant. I liked the sound of that. He clearly explained all the options, allowing me to make the best decision for *me*. In 2007, I began to take Velcade, along with the Zometa.

For the next four years my disease remained relatively stable. Then, in early 2011, after my numbers had begun a slow march upward, Dr. Berenson suggested we add Medrol, a type of steroid, to the mix, and it seems that it was just the boost I needed. As I write this, my numbers are lower than they've been in four years. I go to Curves several days a week, work hard at home on our 20 acres, and feel absolutely great. I had a bit of an adventure last year when, while vacationing in Mexico, my right femur broke spontaneously. All signs indicate that this was due to nine years of Zometa. I've learned this side effect is fairly rare but I have now stopped taking the Zometa per Dr. Berenson's recommendation. Notably, pathology results of a bone sample removed from the fracture site showed no myeloma involvement.

The message I want to send to anyone reading this—patient, family member, caregiver, friend of a patient, or whomever—is that this disease is not a death sentence! I am proof that multiple myeloma can be managed and that quality of life can be wonderful. In my view there are three absolute necessities: (1) An excellent doctor who you trust and who is well-versed in all the latest therapies and is adept at matching them with his patients; (2) A positive "I can do this" attitude on the part of everyone involved, especially the patient; and (3) A good support system, whether it be family, friends, or a "support group." Beyond that, be knowledgeable about your particular disease, keep records of *everything*, and be your own advocate.

I feel so incredibly lucky. In the past ten years, we've been blessed with four more grandkids and countless life-enriching experiences. In May of 2011, I was healthy enough to walk a half marathon to raise money for research for a cure for myeloma. I wish I had the opportunity to talk with every newly-diagnosed patient, because I know how scary it is. It would be my joy and privilege to encourage folks to have hope. The length of survival has been greatly increased, as you can see by reading this book. We all have ups and we all have downs. I would not have wished this illness on myself…or anybody! But it's important to not give up, to move forward and confront it. This is doable.

I Have WHAT???

By Marian S. -- MULTIPLE MYELOMA?!!

Age: 70s

Retired Teacher

I hope the telling of "my journey" gives you hope, encourages you to stay positive and to learn to draw on your source of inner strength, and makes your journey easier. If you are reading this, you or a loved one has just received the most frightening news—if it's presented to you the way it was by my doctor. "You have a terminal illness, and looking at you now, I'd say you have about two to four years to live."

This was over nine years ago; needless to say that doctor didn't know what he was talking about, so don't listen to that kind of talk from anyone! My story began when I was shaving my left leg and noticed the outside had a spot that had no feeling; later I would learn that's called neuropathy. Four doctors each told me, "It's nothing, don't worry about it," so I saw a fifth who took more tests and told me I should see an oncologist because my IgA protein was a little high. He told me not to worry, as that could be quite normal in older people. I was 65 at the time. The oncologist told me I had multiple myeloma. I asked, "What is that?" and he told me, in very few words, about the disease and that I had two to five years to live. He sent us out of his office with an appointment for three months later and not one piece of information on the disease.

My husband Glen and I drove home in shock with little conversation between us, each processing this information. We drove to a park near our home. It was a beautiful March day. We sat on a bench in that small beautiful park filled with flowers, shade trees, and ponds under the beautiful blue sky, holding hands, and looking at God's beautiful creation. I came to my senses and said to Glen, "I am His creation and only He knows my time frame." I called the doctor's office, made an appointment to talk to him and told him why I could not be his patient, and my journey began.

A top priority was to educate myself about the disease from a reliable resource. For me, that was the International Myeloma Foundation (IMF), which holds seminars around the country. Fortunately, there was one scheduled in a few months that was only a five-hour drive from my home. While I waited, I chose a local oncologist and continued to learn more about this disease I had never heard of before.

Attending the seminar was the best gift I could give myself. Myeloma specialists from around the country gave presentations and so much wonderful information was given. I was beginning to feel empowered. The most important of the information was to have a multiple myeloma specialist head my health care team, not just a community oncologist that treats all cancers. This is such a complicated disease to deal with, and this particular cancer is a full-time job to keep current on. Remember, each of us needs an individualized treatment; so much harm can be done to us with a "do it by-the-book" treatment.

On my next doctor visit, I shared this information with him, being very careful with my wording so he would not be offended by this. But despite my attempts to tread lightly, he was. The doctor said he was quite capable of treating my disease, and that I did not need a specialist. Remembering to be my own advocate (something I learned at the seminar), I said I was serious and needed his cooperation. He wasn't very nice about it but relented and gave me the name of a doctor. He said, "If you insist, I will give you the name of the very best multiple myeloma specialist, not just in California, but in the whole country, Dr. James R. Berenson. He is right here in Los Angeles and he has his own research lab."

Little did I know how God had blessed me again when I made that appointment. Dr. Berenson provided me with such hope that I would be living a number of years filled with quality time, due to the many combinations of drugs he could use. More were being researched and would be available down the line. He was not only brilliant but was also kind, loving, caring, sensitive, and provided an atmosphere of calm and openness that made it so easy to talk to him, and he listened.

When we left his office and got into our car, I shed tears of joy and relief that this man would be with me to my journey's end WHICH BEYOND A DOUBT WOUD BE YEARS DOWN THE ROAD. My dear husband felt the same way. Since so much of our life was now going to be in our doctor's office, we didn't want settle for anything but the best. You owe it to yourself, and you will know when you are with the right doctor.

I was fortunate to be diagnosed early as I was in the smoldering stage. It was wait-and-watch with monthly blood tests and treatments of Aredia, a bone strengthener that was administered in a three-hour infusion. Now I take Zometa and it only takes 30 minutes. Of course, I wanted to attack the cancer RIGHT NOW but Dr. Berenson gave me all the information I needed as to why not, and I became quite comfortable with wait-and-watch. I had chosen to treat my myeloma as a chronic disease, with the drugs that were necessary at the time, instead of a stem cell transplant.

Something I dealt with at the beginning was not "Why me?" but "Lord, what do you want me to do with this?" The answer was very clear: When I started chemotherapy I would volunteer for clinical trials, make my contribution as others have done before me, and Glorify Him through my whole journey.

I was blessed with not needing chemotherapy during the first three years and only the monthly treatment with the bone strengthener. I tucked the myeloma in the back of my mind and went on with my busy life. I spent precious time with family, enjoying my young great-grandchildren, traveling with Glen, volunteering with my church, and other normal daily activities. I did notice the sky seemed bluer, flowers were brighter colors than ever before, and little things no longer bothered me. Don't waste a moment, live each day to the fullest.

After coming out of the smoldering stage after three years, my chemotherapy started and was very successful at controlling the myeloma. After that therapy no longer worked, I started the first of my six clinical trials. The papers I had to sign for the protocols were filled with information, I had *lots* of questions, and Dr. Berenson answered them with great patience each time. They came with many side effect that certainly were not always easy, but lots of good results, Dr. Berenson learning from each one. Looking back after each trial I would think, "I'm glad it's over, but I can do that again!" I knew I was in great hands with Dr. Berenson watching me closely, and my faith sustained me through all of it because I knew the Lord was watching over me. For me, that was a "winning combination!"

The last trial has brought me two years of full remission with maintenance treatment. Now my IgA numbers are moving around but still low enough to be in the normal range, and my maintenance therapy continues. I am always confident Dr. B will have something else for me when this no longer works. I have complete confidence he will be involved when the "cure" is found, and it will be! Don't ever give up hope.

At the IMF seminar, I met Gary from my area. We both felt the way to live this myeloma journey would be walking others through support and education. There was not a myeloma patient support group in our area or surrounding areas so we formed one. There were four of us and four caregivers who met at a local restaurant over breakfast. Glen and Roberta (Gary's wife) were great supporters, helping us every step of the way. Over eight years later, our attendance has grown and now averages 30 to 35 people each month who are walking through the journey together. Dr. Berenson and various staff members have given presentations numerous times. They lovingly share their expertise and time.

I have made many great friends in my support group and in the clinic setting. We encourage each other; celebrate the success of a treatment, etc. I am inspired by them; they are some of the most courageous and strongest people I have ever met.

I am thankful for the blessing of Dr. Berenson and his staff, the opportunity to share my story with you, the love and support of my family and friends, and a loving husband willing to drive the freeway in heavy traffic, sitting through hours of clinical trials and chemo treatments with me.

We all will have different stories but our common bond can be to get used to and accept our "new normal" and CHOOSE TO BE HAPPY with the precious time we have.

I Have WHAT???

By Marjorie L. -- MULTIPLE MYELOMA?!!

Age: 60s

Project Manager

I can still remember the phone call. It was in November 1993. My hematologist called me during my four-month-old son's morning nap. I had been feeling pretty ill for over two years, not myself at all for about three or four. I had been to several specialists, even to Scripps Hospital in San Diego for a complete work-up. I was 40 years old, with exhaustion and severe headaches as my symptoms. I saw several neurologists and hematologists over a period of three years. My sed rate was very weird and elevated, my white count low, and I was slightly anemic. But not one doctor could give me a definite diagnosis. I was diagnosed with everything from fibromyalgia to lupus. One doctor even diagnosed me with a very rare disease called Tolosa-Hunt Syndrome and wanted to do brain surgery. Thank God I went to another doctor.

I had gotten pregnant in late 1992. My pregnancy caused severe pain in my lower spine. I was also constantly exhausted during the pregnancy and told that I was almost 40 years old and what did I expect? My son, Kevin, was born in July 1993. I went to my GP soon after and he decided that my blood work was odd enough to send me to a hematologist. He immediately diagnosed me with lupus and started treating me. When I had no response at all he did a battery of tests, including autoimmune ones.

That is when I got the call. "You need to see an oncologist."

"An oncologist, what for?"

"You have cancer. A rare cancer named multiple myeloma."

I was home, with my seven-year-old daughter Courtney at school, and my baby sleeping in his crib. Needless to say, I freaked. The first call was to my GP, who was also a family friend. He was at home that day. When I told him what my diagnosis was, he said that was impossible and he would call my hematologist himself. He called me right back and wanted Mike's (my husband) phone number at work.

Mike came home right away. But first, he stopped at the local library and looked up multiple myeloma. He made a copy of the article he found and brought it home. I was *so* grateful, because the first line of the article said basically that multiple myeloma was a terminal cancer with a life expectancy of three to five years after diagnosis. I could not believe it and refused to believe it.

I knew soon that it was going to take three things to beat this: a positive attitude, lots of moral and spiritual support, and the right doctor. Finding the third proved to be the most difficult and most important of the three.

My husband is one of the most positive and optimistic persons you could meet. He immediately had me thinking correctly. Telling my family wasn't that difficult because I had been sick for a while. There was relief in finally having a diagnosis. Not exactly the diagnosis anyone wanted, though.

Our church immediately kicked into gear and my Bible Study leader set up a Thursday morning prayer and support group at my house. The first week we had six women. Within a month we had over twenty. It was tremendously uplifting. We eventually established a cancer support group at the Church for anyone with any type of cancer. We had eighteen people show up at the first meeting. Eventually, the group ended when I was the only one left. Sadly, the rest had all passed away over a period of about ten years.

The journey to get to Dr. Berenson was interesting. I went to my first oncologist within a week of my wonderful phone call. She was a local oncologist who had a practice and worked with City of Hope. She initially ran some additional tests. She did a bone marrow biopsy and had X-rays done of all the important bones of my body. When we met with her for the results, she said my IgG was 9,600, and my bone marrow biopsy came back at 98% cancer cells. She then diagnosed me with MGUS because she said the X-rays showed no bone involvement. She believed this because the journal she read said that multiple myeloma was found mostly in men in their 70s and included bone involvement. Since I was female, only 40, and had no bone involvement, in her opinion, I did not have cancer.

Of course, this was exactly what we wanted to hear. My husband was ecstatic. I had some real doubts. I wanted a second opinion. I had been reading a book on cancer. The appendix of this book contained support groups for various different cancers. One listing was the International Myeloma Foundation. I called the number given and talked to a wonderful woman named Susie Novis. I told her what my original oncologist had said about my having MGUS. She asked me for my counts which I then read to her. She then asked me if I would mind if she talked to a doctor and then call me back. I was very grateful for her and any knowledgeable person's input at this point. I received a phone call within 30 minutes from an oncologist from Cedars-Sinai Hospital. He asked me to come out the next day for some additional tests and to see him.

My husband and I spent the next day at Cedars. I was poked, prodded, and X-rayed. The sad result was that I had full-blown myeloma, not MGUS. He recommended that I start treatment immediately and gave me some names in Pasadena, much closer to home.

The second oncologist immediately started me on melphalan. It didn't work. He then switched me to VAD (vincristine, Adriamycin, and dexamethasone). This did nothing but make me lose my hair and get very sick. By then, I was desperate. I had absolutely no confidence in this idiot either. My friend was an RN who was working in Home Health. She suggested that I go see a local oncologist named Doug Blayney. During my first appointment, he made a phone call to a friend of his from medical school at Stanford. This friend of Dr. Blayney's was at UCLA at that time and worked almost exclusively with multiple myeloma. His name was James Berenson. This recommendation saved my life. I strongly believe that.

My travels with Dr. Berenson have been long, sometimes tortuous, sometimes scary, but always beneficial. My first appointment was in late 1994, I believe. He took me off of all chemotherapy, even though my IgG was at around 10,000. This was because he wanted me to have a stem cell transplant. You could not have a stem cell transplant if you had 12 cycles of chemotherapy. I had already had 11.

What came next was what caused me to realize that this journey to stay alive was going to require a lot of hard work, and would only work if I became an advocate for myself. I AM MY OWN BEST ADVOCATE. That became my mantra. That is also what I tell every cancer patient I know. No one will fight harder for you to live than you. Fight everyone who says no to treatment, help, or whatever your doctor says you need.

Dr. B. immediately prescribed the stem cell transplant. He told us then that he thought I had drug-resistant multiple myeloma because I had no response to the earlier two chemo regimens. He wasn't sure if the stem cell would work, but he knew chemo wasn't working, so it was my only hope. So, his staff got to work with our insurance company to obtain approval for this procedure.

The insurance company, being what it was, responded with "no" as their first, second, and third response. At this time, the insurance company stated that a stem cell transplant was "an experimental procedure for multiple myeloma." My church group started to see if a way could be found to raise the money to pay for the transplant without insurance. I decided to take a different tact. My husband's company is basically self-insured and the insurance company merely manages the process. So we decided to let the corporate people in New Jersey know what was happening here in California. I called the head of human resources in New Jersey. I had him get to know me. I told him that I had two small children and deserved every chance to see them grow up. I learned how to be my own best advocate. At the end of the day, I got my stem cell transplant, paid in entirety by the insurance company.

My stem cell transplant was scheduled at the end of May 1996. Now came all the stuff you had to do to have the procedure. First, they put a central line in my chest that I swear was as big as a garden hose. This was to be used to collect my stem cells. So, we started to collect.

Every day, my Daddy would drive me to UCLA. Keep in mind, UCLA was almost 50 miles from my house. I came to treasure this time with my Dad, especially since he passed away in 2010. I honestly thought that he would outlive me, and the long drive became very special. I know it was to him also.

I was then told that after 14 days of collection that they hadn't been able to collect enough clean stem cells. So, they then collected them from my hip in a very painful procedure. They still were only able to collect 70% of what they needed for my transplant. But Dr. B. assured me that was enough. He told me my myeloma number was very high (IgG at 14,000), because it took so long to get the procedure approved. He said that they would try to collect enough for two transplants in case of failure. He told me they definitely had enough for one. We obviously knew what we had to pray for at this point.

My stem cell transplant was no walk in the park. I got very sick, developing a high fever. So high in fact the hospital called my husband. They told him that I may not make it and he needed to get to UCLA. But, I surprised them all. I went home the end of June 1996. I was now under Dr. Blayney's care at home due to the distance to Dr. B.'s office. I was home for a week before I was back in the hospital in the Intensive Care unit because I could not keep food down of any kind. This was when I remember thinking that I may not make it after all. But, I surprised everyone, including myself. Three weeks later, I was home and finally recovering.

My IgG went down to 2,000 as a result of my stem cell transplant. It stayed within 500 points of 2,000 for 12 years, never going higher than 2,500 or lower than 2,000. This period was great except for one major problem—NEUROPATHY. It started very suddenly in my left foot in 1997, and advanced very rapidly. I had foot drop within a year and went from using a cane to using a walker very quickly. I saw several neurologists and tried several medications, with nothing working. One neurologist and a highly respected orthopedist that Dr. B had recommended suggested I start walking. They felt that walking might prevent progression of the neuropathy. So I started walking daily. This identified another problem. I had a bad right knee from an injury playing college softball in 1972. So, I had a knee replacement in 2000. I was also diagnosed with Stage 1 uterine cancer in early 2001 and had a radical hysterectomy. Hopefully, that will be my last, final diagnosis with cancer.

The only problem left preventing me from being back to normal was my huge weight gain from the steroids that Dr. Berenson had me taking from 1996 to 2000. He then decided to take me off of them. So, in 2001, I had gastric bypass surgery. Now I was ready. I started walking to prevent the neuropathy from getting worse and to keep the weight off. For eight years, I walked every day from three to five miles. I had an AFO (plastic brace) on my left leg, my walker, and my dog. Every day I love life. I was so grateful to God and Dr. Berenson for giving me my hope and my health back. Initially, I prayed to live long enough to see my daughter graduate from high school. I witnessed this glorious event in 2005. Now, I was praying to get her through college.

I became obsessive about my myeloma and what I could do to keep it where it was. To this day I take vitamin supplements and calcium and try to eat as healthily as I can while still enjoying life as an Italian (who loves food, like all Italians). But in the summer of 2008, I fell walking. I picked myself up and finished another two miles. My hip started to hurt. The next day, I was miserable. I finally went to the ER two days after the fall and found I had broken my hip. Because of the radiation I had earlier and the type of break it was, no surgery was done. I had to spend four to six weeks in bed.

Sometime later, I snapped three bones in my foot. A couple of months after that, I broke two ribs. Then sometime later I broke three more ribs. Ten bones in a little over a year. My myeloma was back. I went out to see Dr. Berenson again and the labs and broken bones told us that the serpent was rearing its ugly head again. He started me immediately on Velcade and dex. That was in mid-2009.

When I broke my hip and couldn't walk my three-mile daily walk, the neuropathy immediately spread to my right foot. By 2009, I was no longer using a walker. I was in a wheelchair. The Velcade didn't help with the neuropathy. The dex was causing a weight gain and water retention. Serious edema developed in both legs. I was still independent even though I was in a wheelchair. The only thing I couldn't do was drive. I was still keeping house, cooking and socializing a lot. I didn't need full time help. I was needlepointing (my hobby and stress reliever). I even started an herb garden on my back patio in elevated pots. The Velcade was slowly but surely working. Dr. Berenson eventually took me off the dex and put me on maintenance Velcade. I would receive treatment only once a month.

Life again became fantastic.

In April 2013, my counts were going up again. When my labs were done on June 13, 2013, they had gone up enough so that Dr. Berenson put me on a different treatment. I started Kyprolis and Treanda in June 2013, with Aloxi to help with the side effect of nausea. I had three full cycles, with the last ending in late August 2013. It worked amazingly. It was very difficult and tiring, but was tolerable because it worked so well. My myeloma number went from 3,240 in June 2013 to 1,640 in August 2013, after only two full cycles! It was GREAT!

In early September 2013, I was transferring from my bed to my wheelchair and fell, snapping my femur in half. This was very surprising to me because I had started bisphosphonate therapy with Aredia in 1994. I continued with the therapy when Zometa was introduced. This therapy was supposed to help strengthen my long bones. I have had almost 20 years of it. Did it fail me? I truly do not know and can only speculate.

It was this break that has changed my life dramatically. I had to undergo surgery. My orthopedist put a rod and pins in my femur. He then told me that I would never be without care again. I was not allowed to put any weight on my leg for three to six months. I went from three weeks in the hospital to two months in a rehab unit. The three to six months ended up being seven months. My bone in the femur was very slow in re-growing.

To this day, I cannot get out of bed or in or out of a car without a Hoyer lift. The neuropathy has completely deadened my bladder and I am 100% incontinent. I have care 24 hours a day now. I am no longer independent. This has been the hardest change I have endured in 21 years of myeloma. It took me seven months to get back to see Dr. Berenson.

We were convinced that my counts would be elevated. I had not finished treatment and in fact, I had had no treatment at all for seven months. I had not even had my correct myeloma labs drawn during this time. I talked to Dr. Berenson for the results of the labs drawn in late March on April 1, 2014, fully expecting him to tell me I had to start treatment immediately. Instead I was told my numbers had only gone up 100 points during those seven months. Again, Dr. Berenson had saved the day (and my life) by prescribing the correct treatment for my myeloma.

Not only have I been alive to see my daughter, Courtney, graduate from high school and college, but my baby boy, Kevin, has also graduated from high school. He has also joined the Army and has a wonderful future ahead of him. I have lived long enough to see both my children become wonderful, productive, loving, and compassionate adults. My husband has stayed by my side through thick and thin. He is an amazing man and I am very lucky to be his wife.

My life has changed a lot during the past 21 years with myeloma. It has not turned out anywhere near what I had planned. But I am alive. My mind is still very bright. I still keep myself as active as possible. All of this is due to the medical care I have received from Dr. Berenson. I am called occasionally by people who live in my area. I always recommend Dr. B., and tell them my longevity is due to my faith in both God and my doctor. And it is also, I believe, due to my positive attitude and the ability to make “lemonade out of lemons.” No matter how bad it is, don't give up. My garden is planted for 2014, and I am needlepointing Christmas gifts.

Remember: Don't let cancer define your life. There is a lot more to you than that.

I Have WHAT???

By Marlene Z. -- MULTIPLE MYELOMA?!!

Age: 70s

Artist

The collage I painted and donated to Dr. Berenson and the Institute for Myeloma & Bone Cancer Research portrays how I imagine the cells in the bone marrow as they change from ominous-looking purple multiple myeloma (MM) cells to healthy cells that are red and pink with a golden background, indicative of their vibrancy following successful treatment of the MM. My life changed when, after having enjoyed wonderful wellness for 64 years, pain began to take over. I was in the midst of completing an important commission from a museum, but I did not want to tell the museum personnel that I was now confined to a wheelchair, for fear they would take away the commission. For months, my husband had to raise and lower the five-by-eight-foot mural in my studio so I could work on it.

On the very day in September 1997 that the museum exhibit was to open with a gala ceremony, featuring my mural in the eight-by-six-by-six-foot Sukkah that I had designed, a wooden structure covered with hundred-year-old grape vines from a local vineyard, I was at my

HMO to hear the results of the tests that I had completed the previous week. I was told I had multiple myeloma!! AND, THEY TOLD ME I NEEDED TO START TREATMENT ON THAT VERY DAY!

My daughter in Beverly Hills told me to get a second opinion, so I postponed the treatment that day and went to the exhibit's debut later that night. At the opening ceremony, I was unexpectedly asked to give a speech about the Sukkah, so I was lifted to the stage in my wheelchair, given a pain pill, and then addressed the several hundred patrons. The mural depicts representative Sukkahs in each state, each located in its proper place on an imaginary US map. After the ceremony, we went to our daughter's home and I learned that she, her husband, a radiologist, and our other children and their spouses had already found out about my diagnosis a few days earlier. They had already made appointments for me to see seven specialists. But my children had already decided who should be my doctor, a world-recognized expert in MM, Dr. James R. Berenson.

He told me that the treatment prescribed by the HMO was not the best one for me and would limit my life span to less than three years. Not only was he optimistic about the possible treatment for me, but also he was an art lover and appreciated my passion for my work. Inspired by his optimism, I decided to embark on the treatment he prescribed: three months of outpatient chemotherapy followed by high doses of chemotherapy and an autologous stem cell transplant in the hospital. I was informed that death was possible, but I did not let that notion stay in my mind. I continued to believe his treatment plan was my best option, so I said, "Let's get on with it."

However, I was not confident that my HMO had enough expertise to provide the care recommended by Dr. Berenson, so I asked the HMO to use him as my doctor. When the HMO refused to do this, I began the process to withdraw from the HMO and to select my own doctor under a different insurance plan. My son, living in New York, coordinated that process by contacting and following up with all of the interested parties. He succeeded and I was able to become a patient of Dr. Berenson's, and I have been under his care to this day.

My myeloma counts started to go down during the outpatient treatment, and the inpatient transplant was then scheduled. My daughter and her husband were major supporters of me during the hospital stay and have been ever since. She made several montages of photos of my grandchildren and placed them around my hospital room on the transplant floor during my three-week stay there. Another daughter who lives in Dallas gave birth to a son while I was still trying to select a doctor, but she (and my son) managed to spend a few nights with me in the hospital a few months later; they and their spouses have been very important sources of help and encouragement ever since.

One scary incident stands out. On the morning that I was to be re-infused with my stem cells that had been collected and frozen weeks earlier, my husband realized that the nurse assigned by UCLA to do the infusion was a trainee; she had never done the procedure before and there was no one assigned to supervise her. In a panic, he phoned Regina, who is Dr. Berenson's head nurse. She, in turn, phoned the charge nurse on our floor, who then agreed to assign an experienced nurse to perform the infusion. However, when the attendant arrived in the room with the frozen stem cells in an ice cart, we discovered that the experienced nurse had left. So, my daughter, who had joined us for the procedure, had to run down the hall to find that nurse and bring her back. The ice-cart attendant warned us that the cells had to be infused within 20 minutes after removal from the cart, or they would spoil. Sure enough, the novice nurse tried but could not do the infusion, so the experienced nurse had to take over.

Incidentally, when UCLA collected my stem cells weeks earlier, I asked them to collect enough to freeze a second bag, but they said their procedure was to collect only one. I have often reflected what could have happened if the one and only bag of cells had been ruined by an inexperienced nurse.

That was 16 years ago. Dr. Berenson says that he now believes that only approximately 3% of his patients have been helped by the transplant procedure that I went through. I have greeted five new grandchildren since then, for a total of eleven. I'm still full of optimism, I work on art every day, and I continue to exhibit and sell my work.

One exciting adventure for me has been to donate art and advice on art for Dr. Berenson's clinic and the Institute for Myeloma & Bone Cancer Research. When he asked me to help design a wall display to depict the financial contributions from donors for the Institute, I devised a metaphor for what they represented. His research is attempting to put together the puzzle that will lead to finding both the causes and cure of multiple myeloma, so I envisioned a display that would reflect that metaphor as a jigsaw puzzle. Each of the interlocking plastic pieces identifies a donor, and the puzzle can be expanded as more contributions are received. This artwork now graces the walls of the Institute and now there is also a smaller version that is displayed in Dr. Berenson's clinic, inspiring patients every day in their quest to discover the cure for patients with multiple myeloma.

I Have WHAT???

By Maureen V. -- MULTIPLE MYELOMA?!!!

Age: Early 60s

Actress and Adult Education Teacher (retired)

Last May, several months after my 60th birthday, I heard a doctor say that I was in his office because it was possible I had multiple myeloma. My regular physician had scribbled "see hematologist" on my results, so I had come for this appointment. I had been anemic before, and thought that some iron pills and a bit more red meat in my diet was about to be prescribed. Instead, the doctor was telling me that there was a good chance I had cancer—me, with my healthy weight, low cholesterol, low blood pressure, and active lifestyle. A bone marrow biopsy confirmed the diagnosis, and a new chapter in my life had begun.

Within several hours after talking with this new doctor, my engineer-scientist husband and I had been on the internet and were aware of the median survival rate and disabling effects of this disease. Needless to say, we were scared, depressed, and not sure how to proceed. I told a good friend what was happening, and she said I should call her friend Jimmy Berenson. I had met Jim and his wife

Debra over 25 years ago, and we occasionally saw each other at Screen Actors Guild Film Society screenings. He and I had spoken about the fact that we both are identical twins. I knew he was an oncologist, but was unaware that his area of expertise was, in fact, multiple myeloma. I called Dr. Berenson and he told me to come in immediately. After another round of intense Googling, my husband and I realized that Dr. B. was an expert in the field of multiple myeloma, involved with the development of new treatments, and that his patients' life spans were above the norm.

I am so lucky to be under the care of a doctor who truly explains things, is focused on the quality of life, answers questions, and quickly returns phone calls. His wonderful and caring staff made visits to the office pleasant and non-frightening.

Now, I am asymptomatic and truly enjoying my life. At first, I had chemotherapy, and when that wasn't as successful as we had hoped, Dr. B. started me on a course of Revlimid and methylprednisone, and the results have been excellent. Last November, I climbed the Great Wall of China!

Nevertheless, multiple myeloma has changed me. I want to do everything right now—travel, hike, tap dance, learn a new language, volunteer, et cetera. I can't help but feel that something bad can happen at any moment so you must enjoy life when you can. And I love my life—this ordeal of multiple myeloma has made me realize how fortunate I am to have a loving husband, wonderful daughter, and great friends and family.

I Have WHAT???

By Maxine J. -- MULTIPLE MYELOMA?!!

Age: 60s

Retired RN

I was diagnosed with MM at age 65, in November 2011. However, I had been experiencing symptoms for several months prior to the diagnosis. It started with pain in my right hip. For several months the doctors at Kaiser thought the pain was due to pulled muscles. As the pain got worse, they finally did the tests that revealed MM. By this time, I was using a walker to get around.

I didn't know anything about MM when I got the bad news. The doctors at Kaiser recommended for me to undergo a stem cell transplant. I didn't feel comfortable with this proposal, and I shared my concerns with my family. Fortunately, my son, Chris, and his wife, Janna, looked at a lot of information on the internet. That's when they found Dr. Berenson. Finding Dr. Berenson was a Godsend for me. We got the first available appointment.

To make a long story short, Dr. Berenson quickly turned my despair to hope. While the Kaiser doctors had been pessimistic, Dr. B. was enthusiastic about my chances. For example, the Kaiser doctors said I was already in Stage 3, but Dr. B. assured me I was barely Stage 1, which lifted my spirits a lot right away.

I appreciated the fact that Dr. B. took the time to study my tests and get to know me personally before developing a personal, customized plan of chemotherapy and other treatments to fight the cancer. It didn't take long for the plan to take hold. Within a few months, the hip pain started to disappear and, eventually, it was totally gone. Today I'm doing yoga and Zumba several times each week.

It's been almost 18 months since I first learned that I had MM. During the first eight months of treatment by Dr. Berenson, my numbers improved significantly and stayed low until this past March when Dr. B noticed a spike, which has resulted in a new series of treatments that have been going on for eight months. While my numbers may have changed, I haven't experienced any new pain or any other problems. I give a lot of credit to my new, improved diet and the regular exercise. I juice a lot more than I ever did before, and I usually start my day with a breakfast of flax seed oil blended with organic cottage cheese. I eat more fruits and vegetables and less meat, and I drink alkaline water on a regular basis.

I would like to thank Dr. Berenson for his MM research team. Because of their research, I am another fortunate soul to live a healthier and happier quality of life. Thank you, Regina, and your excellent nursing staff who make me feel so well cared for. I feel like

I belong to this special happy family of understanding and compassion.

From day one when I met you, I felt very welcome and you filled me with hope for my future with this mysterious MM. Yes, you, "Miss" Barbara at the front desk, thank you for all that you do for me and other patients.

This journey of MM has strengthened my faith in Jesus Christ. I stand healed by His promises and at His timing. MM has taught me how truly precious and beautiful life is and I have no fear of death. I am very optimistic about my future. My wonderful husband and family are immeasurable supports to me. It is all good. And I pray Dr. Berenson and his team find the "cure" in the near future.

I Have WHAT???

By Phyllis G. -- MULTIPLE MYELOMA?!!

Age: 73

Retired Teacher and Paralegal

My New Abnormal. Yes, that is what I call this season of life. It is not normal. It is not healthy. I do not embrace it, welcome it, or like it. "Dr. Berenson, get this beast out of my body!" Am I angry or in denial? No, paradoxically, quite to the contrary. In this journey with Multiple Myeloma, I have encountered the Truth, and have been empowered and enriched beyond imagination.

About four years ago, one of my knees had been bothering me to the point that I was scheduled for knee replacement surgery. However, deep inside, uncertainty nagged. How can I possibly undergo major surgery when I feel so tired? I have no inner "oomph." And why do I feel not just tired, but profoundly fatigued? I am healthy. I am not a tired personality. Yet after an appointment with my internist in Santa Barbara, I had to crawl into the back of my SUV to take a nap to restore enough energy to make the short, 30-mile return trip back to my home in Ventura. That was not normal. And, indeed, it was not for me. Pre-op blood results disclosed that I was seriously anemic.

But why? Many tests later produced the definitive, out-of-the-blue diagnosis: Multiple Myeloma. That did not sound good. What's that? I did not have a clue. And thus, began the fascinating, amazing, and rewarding journey.

After undergoing numerous further tests, I was referred to another doctor who was an internist, hematologist, and oncologist, all wrapped up in one capable, experienced, dedicated physician. Suzie Cream Cheese here waltzed into his office (more like stumbled), thanking him for seeing me and expressing appreciation for his internal medicine and hematology skills, but that I, thankfully, did not need oncology services. But by this time, I felt terrible. "Crappy" was my word for it. In fact, I knew that I was quickly and quietly slipping away . . . dying. It was peaceful, but I did not want to die, and I was frustrated beyond my limits of frustration. Prior tests had been accomplished only with lengthy delays and what seemed like interminable, flimsy excuses. By now it was the day before Thanksgiving 2014, and I was pissed . . . and even rude. Apologizing for my rudeness, I said "Doctor, I need help and I need it now. I am dying, and I don't care what holiday it is or what other people's schedules or plans are. I need help now!" Looking me straight in the eye and with kindness, he said "I am going to help you, and I am going to help you now." With that, he picked up the phone to the lab across the street and said, "I am sending you a patient, now, and I want this, this, and this test done . . . now."

Tests were done, and then The Verdict. Oops. Major problem. Multiple Myeloma. Suzie Cream Cheese melted. And now to consider choices of how to handle it. Having great confidence in this capable doctor, I was agreeable to beginning treatment in Santa Barbara under his guidance. At the same time, I suggested that if, with his vast contacts, he knew of any resources within the U.S. that he felt would be appropriate for my situation, I would be interested to know of them. With that, he picked up the phone once again. That call was to James Berenson, MD at the Institute for Myeloma & Bone Cancer Research in West Hollywood. "Jim, I have a patient who I think will qualify and benefit from your Elotuzumab trial."

After meeting with Dr. Berenson and after more tests at his clinic, I did indeed qualify and began treatment on January 15, 2015 . . . feeling horrible and very much not like my usual healthy self. Infusions began at the rate of once a week for the first eight weeks, followed by every other week after that. At one point, I was hastily rushed to nearby Cedars-Sinai Medical Center for a transfusion of three units of blood because my hemoglobin was dangerously low. At first, I thought infusion treatments would be for a certain period of time and then would end. Not with MM. There is no cure, yet, for MM. So, treatments have continued and will continue . . . for life, or until there is a cure. It is now considered to be a chronic disease, treatable but not curable. That was a bit of an adjustment to accept!

But the day of all days in my journey was the day of the first infusion . . . January 15, 2015. Growing up in Southern California, I was an outdoor girl . . . camping, hiking, horseback riding, swimming, tennis . . . healthy, and from three generations of capable doctors in the family, grandfather, father, and brother. We all do health, not sickness. But here I was, sitting in the waiting room of Dr. Berenson's office, waiting to go down the hall to my first infusion. I was so petrified that I couldn't even turn my head to look down the hall to The Room.

Despite having gone to college in the 1960s, I never had done drugs. Take anything out of me, but don't put toxic drugs into me! I was between a rock and a hard spot: I don't want the drugs, but if I don't have them, I'll die. And I don't want to die. Jesus Lord, please help me. I am in trouble. I don't feel I can do this on my own. I can't get my feet to work. I can't walk down that hall. I just can't do toxic drugs. And then, something completely unanticipated and extraordinary happened. In the midst of my silent caterwauling, boom! Jesus appeared right in front of me.

Yes, I am a Christian believer, but Jesus standing right in front of me?!! Everything faded in the presence of this glorious Being, shining in white robes, tall, strong, commanding, magnificent . . . silent . . . with only the office fish tank in the background behind Him. I could not make out His face, but captivating strength and power emanated from Him. I was startled and stunned into silence of my own. Not a word was spoken. I was riveted by Him. And powerfully, with no words spoken, I received His clear messages of assurance. The messages came in four, distinct parts:

(1) "Phyllis,"

(2) "I love you,"

(3) "I have you in the palm of My hand,"

(4) "I will be with you every step of the way."

With that, He gently faded from my awareness. Breathless, I realized that every part of His assurance was intensely personal and scriptural. Of course, He's God. He speaks only The Truth:

(1) He called me by name. "The Lord knows those who are his." (2 Tim 2:19),

(2) He said He loves me. "He who loves me will be loved by my Father, and I too will love him and show myself to him." (John 14:21),

(3) He said He holds me in His hand. "If the Lord delights in a man's way, he makes his steps firm; though he may stumble, he will not fall, for the Lord upholds him with his hand." (Ps 37:23-24), and

(4) He will be with me. "I will never leave you nor forsake you." (Jos 1:5)

I then stood up and, with strength not of my own, I walked down the hall to the infusion room for the first treatment. That was 72 infusions ago, and counting.

How has it been possible to cope with a deadly cancer for which there is presently no cure? As you can tell by now, faith has played a major role. Having a positive attitude and being consistent and diligent with treatment are also essential. Some friends have asked me to write a book, which I may do one day, perhaps. If I were to write it today, I think the title would be *Gratitude in the Journey: The Art of Suffering*. I am grateful that my case was diagnosed as early as it was. I am grateful for competent doctors who were able to make a correct diagnosis. I am especially grateful for the referral to Dr. Berenson and the IMBCR.

Working directly with Dr. B, who is one of the most competent and knowledgeable physicians in the field, is key. A general oncologist simply will not do, no matter how well-intentioned. It gives me great confidence to know that Dr. B watches everything about my case. I know in my "knower" that he would call me if there were concerns of any sort. Nothing slips by him. He knows what is appropriate for me. He provides his cell number to his patients, and he answers e mails promptly. If his staff does not know the answer to a question, they find out and get back to the patient. His entire organization, from the top down, is remarkable. It is actually a pleasure to go to the Institute, even though the numerous trips are time-consuming and inconvenient. Where can a patient meet face to face with a high-caliber, dedicated, caring, generous, competent specialist (one of the best in the world!), have a hands-on physical exam, and a complete blood panel before each infusion . . . every two weeks!

No wonder I look healthy and well, and people say they would never know I have a serious disease. In his own research labs and with his connections with the best and brightest around the world, Dr. Berenson is in the know regarding advances in treatment, and he is at the forefront of progress in the search for a true cure. As I tell him, we are going straight from my current, effective treatment to the cure.

Meanwhile, Dr. B has provided me with the opportunity to continue to live, probably for many years to come, and to live with a good quality of life. And for that I am profoundly grateful. Yes, the disease process has been arrested for the time being and yes, there are unpleasant side effects to some of the meds. My immune system is basically non-functional, which places me at risk of infections. And I have had some. I have digestive issues as a result of Revlimid. I fatigue easily. I bruise easily and have other medication-related symptoms: blurry vision, dizziness, "highs" from Dex. And I have elevated risk factors for other diseases. But all of those things are manageable with some alterations in lifestyle.

And perhaps most encouraging of all to me are the many, many people who know of my journey and who say, "You give us such hope." "You are such an encouragement." That encourages me! To be an encouragement to others is a profound honor. I find support groups depressing, so I don't go. I don't want to hear all the awful things that could happen to me. Instead, I am living. I am thriving. I am grateful. And in the suffering that goes along with the process, if I can provide another with the courage and enough knowledge about this disease to persevere towards the cure, well, it's all worth it.

What would I say to someone newly diagnosed with MM? Don't despair. Get into treatment right away with someone like Dr. B so you can continue to enjoy your life and can be part of the solution at the IMBCR, as we push towards the cure so there will one day be no more patients suffering from MM!

I Have WHAT???

By Robert D., MD -- MULTIPLE MYELOMA?!!

Age: 60s

Psychiatrist

My back was hurting. A lot. In March 2010, I suddenly developed severe lower back pain. For a few days, I could barely move. Oh well, I told myself—lots of people get back pain. Most of my friends have suffered from this. I took ibuprofen, aspirin, Tylenol, and when it was really bad, some Vicodin. A few days later the pain decreased, and I was able to get around reasonably well, even though my back still hurt a lot. A month or so later the pain suddenly increased again. And then it happened again so I hobbled around. I took more medication, and I managed somehow. I was also really tired. Well, pain makes people tired, doesn't it? One friend told me to see a chiropractor (I didn't); another said get physical therapy (I did). After three weeks of treatment, the physical therapist said, "You aren't getting better, so maybe you should see a back specialist . . ." So I went to Dr. P., a well-respected orthopedist. The office visit lasted no more than two minutes (really!). After a 15-second exam he said: "Well you probably have a disk problem. I'll send you for an MRI, and come back in a week." A week later, on June 17, 2010, I was back in his office. He put the MRI up on the viewing box and told me "You have three compression fractures. It looks like they are from metastatic cancer; you should see an oncologist." No wonder I had so much pain. That time the visit lasted one minute longer than my first time there—three minutes.

I called an oncologist, Dr. Gary Cecchi, whom I know well; we are colleagues at Alta Bates Medical Center in Berkeley. He told me to come to his office right away. I got in the car and set off driving. And I called my wife. After gasping about the news, she said she would meet me at Dr. Cecchi's office. She arrived not long after I was sitting in his office. Dr. Cecchi said he would perform a bone marrow biopsy right then and get a PET scan. He told me we'd probably know the diagnosis very soon. By the next day, the diagnosis did come back—multiple myeloma. I am a physician, but I didn't know a lot about myeloma. What I remembered wasn't good—I recalled that this kind of cancer is incurable and that people who get it die a painful death within a few years of being diagnosed. But, Dr. Cecchi told me that things have changed a lot for the better, and that I was likely to do very well. He told me to come back the next week for my first dose of chemotherapy. He also told me that he is a general oncologist and that I should get a consultation with an expert in the field; he recommended Dr. James Berenson in Los Angeles. He also told me: "You are going to have some tough decisions to make." I didn't know what he meant, but I called Dr. Berenson's office for an appointment and went there two and a half weeks later.

I did a lot of reading. I learned that in fact this disease can be well controlled. I also learned that many people were being treated with autologous peripheral blood stem cell transplants. Now I knew what Dr. Cecchi meant when he said I'd have some decisions to make.

The drive to LA was pretty bad. I was in a lot of pain whenever I moved even a little. Just getting out of bed was a challenge; so was getting dressed. Dr. Berenson was as thorough as Dr. P. was cursory. He took a complete history and did a very thorough physical exam. He asked me if I had any pain, tingling, or numbness and I said a little in my fingers. I was already getting peripheral neuropathy from the chemotherapy, even though I only had received a few doses. He revised my regimen, reducing the dose of Velcade and lengthening the cycle from three to four weeks, and making some other changes as well. With the new dose and longer cycle of Velcade, the numbness in my fingers went away. I'm an amateur guitarist and bass player —I was so glad I could feel the tips of my fingers again!

Dr. Berenson said my back pain should have been addressed weeks earlier; he called a neurosurgical colleague on the phone. The surgeon had just gotten off a plane from India but was willing to see me that afternoon. My wife and I went there and learned that balloon kyphoplasty was a procedure that could provide impressive pain relief. All this was happening boom, boom, boom. I could hardly believe it, especially after the so-called care I had received from Dr. P. Within a week I underwent a kyphoplasty—two days after that, the pain was much better, and it continued to decrease as the weeks went by. The procedure did not restore the 1½-inch loss of height that I had experienced, but it gave me pain relief, and I guess it must have stabilized the affected vertebrae.

Like Dr. Berenson, I am a thorough kind of guy—I saw three other myeloma experts, one at UCSF, one at the Mayo Clinic in Scottsdale, Arizona, and one at the Dana-Farber Cancer Institute in Boston. Two of the three doctors recommended a stem cell transplant, but the third said it was a toss-up. Both Drs. Cecchi and Berenson told me that I would probably do just as well or better without a transplant, and they explained the biological and clinical information that led them to their recommendation for me not to undergo that form of treatment. In the end, I decided to forgo the transplant.

I'm glad—I'm doing really well. I finished my initial course of treatment with Velcade, Doxil, and dexamethasone, which was based on laboratory work followed by a clinical trial that Dr. Berenson conducted. It's now seven and a half years since I was diagnosed with multiple myeloma. There have been setbacks that have required changes in my medications but so far, I am winning, not the myeloma. A few years ago, I had increased back and neck pain and learned that the disease was attacking the vertebral bones in my back and neck again. I had additional kyphoplasties and my myeloma meds were changed.

Now my most recent duration of controlling the disease has been for close to a year. Each time the myeloma attacks we fight back and we have been successful every time. At present, I have an infusion of medication every week or so. It hasn't been a problem. I sit in the comfortable reclining chair and read or listen to music.

I should add that I have an unusual form of myeloma called "non-secretory," in which no myeloma protein levels can be detected. Only a small percentage of myeloma patients are non-secretory. It makes my disease harder to track; progress can be determined by PET scans, bone marrow biopsies, and a new test that Dr. Berenson has developed—measuring the amount of a protein called BCMA in my blood. The results of all of these tests have been very good. Although I have not been cured, the level of myeloma activity is low.

My wife and I travel to Los Angeles every three months to see Dr. Berenson. He devises the treatment strategy and Dr. Cecchi implements the plan here at home. This treatment has been successful. I hardly have any side effects. I am working and I am enjoying life—family, friends, travel, and my music. I don't feel like a cancer patient. I can do almost anything; I can walk ten miles without much difficulty and I'm nearly 75. My wife and I just got back from a vacation in Paris—we walked all over, went to museums, ate lots of good food and just basked in the beauty we saw all around us.

The visits to Dr. Berenson's office are enjoyable. My wife and I drive the six hours from Northern California to Los Angeles and make the trip a mini-vacation. It's fun seeing Dr. B and I never feel that he is rushing through my appointments with him. He has the uncanny ability to be friendly and personal as well as professional. The folks in his office are also wonderful—kind, attentive, and caring at all times.

My family and friends have also been vitally involved. I have read about the power of love and how love can heal. Now I have experienced it. Friends and family members have been there throughout the process, sometimes a little and sometimes a lot. No one has done so much as my wife, Margarita. I appreciated her a lot before I got sick but now much, much more. She has been with me all through the process and makes sure everything that can promote my health is being done. Let me tell you, all she needs to do is look at me and I feel better.

I know a lot about myeloma now. It is still a terrible disease, but with modern care and also with some luck I know that it is a disease I can live with, hopefully for many, many years, with good fortune, love, and excellent medical care until I die of something else. I have had wonderful people who have helped me and are still there for me—my wife, my children, Dr. Cecchi and his staff, and Dr. Berenson and his staff. What would I have done without them?

I Have WHAT???

By Roger T. -- MULTIPLE MYELOMA?!!

Age: 60s

CPA; Avocado Farmer; Real Estate Developer

Eight years ago, I had my annual physical and my doctor told me that my red blood cell count had dropped well below normal. I had been taking iron supplements because my red blood cell count had been low for the past year or two. He sent me back for a few more tests and found that my blood and urine protein levels were too high. He recommended that I have a bone marrow biopsy. I was referred to a local oncologist to review the results.

I knew that something must be up; why else would my doctor send me to an oncologist?

I wasn't prepared for the answer. The oncologist bluntly told me that I had an incurable and deadly cancer called "multiple myeloma." I responded with: "What was that?" He said that it was a type of blood and bone cancer. I had never heard of it! How could this be? I have always been healthy and active and now I had a cancer that could end my life!

Through researching, I found out that there was no known cure for multiple myeloma… Now my head was really spinning! Being a calculating person (a CPA) I realized that the odds of getting this disease were 100,000 to one. More common than I would have thought. What a bummer; God sure wasn't on my side!

I searched my mind as to how I could have been diagnosed with cancer; no one in my family had this type of disease. But, then I read and realized that there seemed to be a higher likelihood of getting this if you came from a farming background. I have a farm business and thought that perhaps I had been exposed to too many chemicals. We used herbicide weed control spray and that could be another factor that caused me to get multiple myeloma. It could be that I grew up in Central America and was exposed to DDT spray (which was used to keep the insects under control).

But, at some point it no longer matters how you get a disease, you just need to deal with the disease you have! So, my wife and I did some research on the web. At first I was reluctant to tell anybody that I had been diagnosed with multiple myeloma. I'm not sure why I felt like that, but I did.

But, when I decided to tell my family and friends, my fortunes began to change as did my outlook. I was very fortunate to have several doctors as friends. As I shared my new situation, it was amazing how many of them offered connections and resources to me.

After a month or so, a surfing buddy of mine knew of a local dermatologist who also had multiple myeloma, so I gave him a call. He was going to a doctor in West Hollywood known to be researching this type of cancer. I decided to contact that doctor and the two of us carpooled to West Hollywood from Orange County.

Well, that doctor was James Berenson, and my life has been blessed ever since. I started treatment in May 2004. I found out that I was in an early phase of myeloma, so my doctor visits and treatments were monthly. I say I was blessed because Dr. Berenson and his staff have consistently cared for my myeloma, and I have been able to live a normal, full life, with reason to believe that I will have many more years to enjoy with my family and friends.

As time went by, my myeloma numbers would go up and Dr. Berenson would change the medication and sometimes I would be part of a clinical trial that he was doing. Also, through the years with Dr. Berenson's treatments, my myeloma numbers would fall to remission levels. I have been in a remission or on maintenance therapy for rest of the time.

I have been on nine different cancer treatment protocols. Each time the drugs have beaten back the bad cells, and on three occasions, I was able to go on to a maintenance treatment for more than a year, and once close to two years. Maintenance therapy is a great place to be because there are little, if any, side effects with the lower dose intensity of the drugs, and the trips to the doctor's office are greatly reduced. The real challenge with myeloma is that those nasty "bad" cells keep finding a way to work around the medication after a while. But, the good thing about having it is that Dr. Berenson is a dedicated researcher and he is always coming up with new combination therapies that can keep things under control.

Over the eight years I've been living with myeloma, I have been able to maintain a normal active lifestyle with Dr. Berenson's help. I operate three businesses (a CPA practice, an avocado farm, and a real estate development company). I've been able to participate in my favorite sports (surfing and skiing) and enjoy many family vacations. Dr. Berenson supports me by scheduling my office visits around my trips when needed. Most of the time, I actually forget that I have anything wrong with me. Isn't that great?!

Throughout the years with my early-morning appointments with Dr. Berenson and his medical staff, a trust has developed. He is one of the most knowledgeable myeloma experts in the world and here he is very close to my home—right here in Southern California! I know that I will be well taken care of and treated with respect and valued as a "whole" person. To find such caring and support from someone who spends much of his time researching is a real gift.

Dr. Berenson is head of the Institute for Myeloma & Bone Cancer Research. His efforts to find a cure and to work with other experts on this form of cancer have been of considerable benefit to my care.

In the eight years that I have had multiple myeloma, I have never once felt that my situation was hopeless. In fact, I'm hopeful every day that some time in my future Dr. Berenson will announce that the battle has been won.

I Have WHAT???

By Ron R. -- MULTIPLE MYELOMA?!!

Late 60s

Public Relations/Public Affairs/Rancher

I've had multiple myeloma (MM) for 17 years, thanks to Dr. Berenson! I was told I would only live three or four years by the first doctor I saw, but boy, was he wrong… I want to keep on trucking.

I would like to say to those newly diagnosed with MM that in the past 17 years, my disease has been nothing more than a minor inconvenience. Only twice, when I had to have chemotherapy, has my course been difficult. I have been able to live life to the fullest. My advice to other people that have been diagnosed with this disease is to "Cowboy up, stop whining, and move on with something you can do."

Other patients in Dr. B.'s clinic ask me what my numbers are. They know their numbers, but I don't know mine. I leave that to Dr. Berenson. There is nothing I can do about my numbers, so I don't want to worry about them. I will say that I do get a little anxious when I am going in for a checkup, though. I hope that I get a good report, and most times things are just fine.

I have been basically a very healthy person. I work in the city in public relations and public affairs, but enjoy getting out of town and going to my ranch in Colorado. I do a lot of heavy work at the ranch, ride horses and ATVs, and have chickens, goats, and all sorts of other animals. I tell Dr. B. that it must be all of that cow manure that is keeping my disease in control.

Before I was diagnosed, I remember when I was taking a hike with one of my good friends and every so often I had to stop to catch my breath. I felt like I was out of air. In retrospect, that was one of the first signs that something was wrong with me.

The other symptom I had was that I started feeling tired at the ranch—granted, the altitude is 7,000 feet, but that had never been a problem before. I was used to working 12-hour days in the hot sun and I probably had twice the energy as most other people.

I go for regular checkups. I went in to see what was going on with me. The doctor gave me a regular exam and took the usual blood tests. He said that everything was just fine and not to worry. But I knew something wasn't right. I wasn't tired just because I was getting older—I just didn't feel like myself.

Finally, during a checkup a few months later, an abnormality did show up in one of my blood tests. That's when the doctor gave me the dreaded news that I had multiple myeloma and that I had only three or four years to live! I thought he said "melanoma"—I had never heard of MM. So I went online, and what I read scared me to death. I think I was in shock. The statistics didn't look too good. But, during my research, I kept seeing Dr. Berenson's name mentioned in many of the articles about MM and learned that he also took care of patients with this problem.

I remember getting away and going out of town to the ranch with my wife, Lisa. I didn't tell her my news until I was able to process it. Then, the only other person I told about my diagnosis was my assistant, Emmy. Her father had recently died of cancer and I wanted to know if she'd be able to hold this information in confidence. Would she be able to help me with the needed doctor appointments and keep my "business as usual" façade up? Because I am in the PR business, I didn't want my diagnosis to affect my business, and I thought that if people found out that I had MM, it would, and not in a good way. I did not want to tell my mother, either. She was older and not well at the time. I knew that my diagnosis would break her heart. So, because of all of these reasons, I chose to tell very few people.

My wife agreed with me that I should see Dr. Berenson and also see the doctor that my regular doctor recommended—I would seek out two opinions. The other doctor said that I needed a stem cell transplant right away or I would die. Then, I went to see Dr. Berenson. He said that he didn't think that I needed a transplant—that I was in good shape and young (I was 55 at the time). He also said that he'd like to put me on a trial with a drug called Zometa, which had not yet been FDA-approved.

I went back to the other doctor just to see why he thought that I needed a transplant. I wanted him to know that Dr. Berenson said that I didn't need one, and would only give me treatment with monthly Zometa as part of a clinical trial since the drug was still experimental at that time. I'll never forget what the doctor said to me: "You better make up your mind which doctor is going to be treating you." I said, "I just did" and I left his office for Dr. Berenson's clinic.

I never did have that stem cell transplant and that was 17 years ago. Dr. B. put me on the Zometa trial and I responded, with my myeloma numbers improving. I felt great on that monthly treatment for eight years. We didn't have to do anything else!

I did try chemotherapy later on at two different occasions. I didn't tolerate it very well either time. Chemo knocked me for a loop. I was happy when I was finished with it.

One time I was at my ranch in Colorado and I felt terrible for a couple of days after starting a new pill to treat my MM. So, I called Dr. B. and he said that I should go right to the local hospital. I saw the doctor there and they took some blood and then I was sent back to the ranch. When I got back, Dr. B. had gotten the results of my blood tests and told me that I needed to go right back to the hospital because I was in kidney failure from that pill, which was an extremely rare side effect. It is so great that Dr. Berenson is always available on his cell phone. He wants his patients to call him if they have a problem, so that they will get the best possible care resulting in improved outcomes for all of his patients.

Besides fatigue, I have experienced neuropathy (numbness, tingling, and fatigue) and occasionally some bone-related problems that are actually not from the multiple myeloma. I also take alpha-lipoic acid for my neuropathy and I take calcium and vitamin D to strengthen my bones.

I have had some bone and kidney issues that may be related to having been on Zometa for such a long period of time. I had a stress fracture in my foot a few years ago. My work at the ranch is strenuous, bad backs run in my family, and I have fallen off of horses and motorcycles more times than I care to remember. I also have a little bit of arthritis in my back. Sometimes I get cortisone injections and that helps.

Once when I was traveling to India, I took an antibiotic called Levaquin. Well, apparently it restricts the function of tendons and stays in your system for a very long time. After returning from India, I got out of bed one morning and pulled my Achilles tendon. Also, I have an intermittent condition called "foot drop" which is related to the neuropathy I developed from some of the myeloma drugs. I have also had balance problems from the neuropathy. I developed some problems in my hip because I couldn't walk normally on my foot. I chose not to have a cap redone on a tooth when in normal circumstances I would have. I am very careful with my teeth because I have had some jaw problems from being on Zometa. But, these problems have not been a big deal for me. Again, the benefits of being on Zometa far outweighed the side effects. So, the dentist just keeps putting in a temporary filling and if it falls out he just puts in a new one again. That way we avoid any significant problems that can exacerbate my jaw issues.

I accompanied Dr. Berenson to the FDA in Washington, DC a few years ago when they were concerned about the jaw problems from Zometa. I testified at the meeting and told them that I was a walking example of a patient doing well because of this drug. Even if there were jaw problems in some patients, they were easily managed in most patients. What was the alternative? Zometa continues to be used and patients are now made aware of ways to reduce the risk of jaw problems—good dental health and avoid having any teeth removed or having dental implants.

I just keep looking for answers and keep on pushing ahead. When the treadmill became difficult for me to use, we traded it for an elliptical machine. At one point, I could only do 5 minutes without stopping and now I can do 20 minutes four or five times every week. I also find creative ways to get onto my horse if I can't get up there the usual way. Sometimes I step on the picnic table to get on or get off in a ditch. I do allow myself to get mad for one minute, but then I simply move on. I find being positive is a lot more productive.

Today, I woke up and found that my toe is probably broken. But, what can you do?

After my mother passed away, I finally decided to tell my family, friends, and business associates that I was living with MM and that it was a chronic disease for me. I wanted to help raise some funds for the Institute for Myeloma & Bone Cancer Research (IMBCR), the non-profit research laboratory entity that Dr. Berenson created to develop new treatments for MM. I became a founding board member of IMBCR and remain so to this day. I was doing very well and I wanted to continue to do well.

I was able to obtain funds from Wallace Annenberg and the Skirball Foundations to help get the Institute up and running. Because I don't like compliments and asking people for money, my friends, Bruce and Toni, decided to have a benefit at their home a few years ago to help raise some of the needed research funds for trials at the Institute.

Also, we were honored to host the inaugural event for the IMBCR at our home in 2004. Because of my wife Lisa's connections with women in politics, Geraldine Ferraro spoke at the event about living with MM and graciously answered questions at a lively Q&A. It was a great event.

It gives me satisfaction to help other people that have MM. I was at the clinic the other day and there was a patient sitting next to me with his head down. I noticed that his wife was trying to cheer him up. I tried to start a conversation with him and asked him how long he has been seeing Dr. Berenson. He said that this was just his second visit. I told him that I had been a patient of Dr. B.'s for 14 years. He picked up his head and I could see that he was much more relaxed. There was hope in his eyes. There is camaraderie among Dr. B.'s patients. We support each other here.

I've never seen a doctor like Dr. Berenson. He is excited describing what are the latest results from experiments he has going on in the Institute's laboratory. He has the passion, curiosity, and the scientific background that makes him a great doctor. He really cares about all of his patients and their quality of life.

I feel very lucky. My life is good. I thought I was going to be dead five or ten years ago and I'm not. I just keep on trucking. My wife and I just celebrated our 30th anniversary and I look forward to many more occasions, fun times at the ranch and interesting PR work. Keep those discoveries coming, Dr. Berenson!

I Have WHAT???

By Stephen & Susan B. -- MULTIPLIE MYELOMA?!!

Age: 60s

Economics Professor and Writer

Stephen

The day after Thanksgiving 2015, I had an appointment that was the beginning of a life-changing experience. I thought I had a routine physical problem, but was told that I needed some additional tests. My general practitioner called me at home and told me I needed to be tested to see if I had multiple myeloma—something I had never heard of. After a series of doctors' visits and tests, I finally had a definitive bone marrow test and I was told by an oncologist where I live that I had multiple myeloma. It took 67 days from the time I started testing until I heard the news.

Even though it seemed like it took forever, those days were important for us. We had time to research and study and find Dr. James Berenson. We searched the internet, and read whatever we could find. We were just trying to get a handle on multiple myeloma and what it meant to have it. And, most importantly when you hear you have cancer, what it meant for my life.

Searching the internet for information on multiple myeloma taught me two things. The first was that there is a lot of bad and out-of-date information out there. The second was that Dr. Berenson in Los Angeles and MD Anderson in Houston had the best outcomes for their patients. I live a few hours from Los Angeles, so I made an appointment with Dr. Berenson even before I knew I had multiple myeloma. That decision changed my life in so many ways.

I wasn't feeling very sick and had no classic symptoms of multiple myeloma. I expected to hear that I had MGUS, but when we found out it was multiple myeloma it was a big shock. A few days after we received the news, we drove to Los Angeles and met Dr. Berenson. He completely turned our world around—he was encouraging, and he let us know that the disease was very treatable and that people can live for many, many years with multiple myeloma. He told us he had many different treatment regimens and that if one wasn't the right fit for me, another one would be. His positive information and attitude gave us so much hope. I also loved the fact that he was a fellow researcher and totally dedicated to erasing multiple myeloma from the earth.

We agreed that he would direct my treatment in conjunction with my oncologist where I live. I receive infusions in my hometown and visit Los Angeles monthly (now every two months) to have Dr. Berenson assess the progress. I've been lucky to have my two-city team and I've been extremely lucky to have responded well to the initial treatment I received. Since diagnosis, I've had multiple myeloma for one year and three months, and I feel and look so much better than when I started treatment.

Finding Dr. Berenson was the key to having what I consider a successful treatment. First, because he put me on a different treatment plan that I would have had from my hometown oncologist. And second, because Dr. Berenson and his caring staff are always there for us. The encouragement from both my doctors and the loving care I receive from the oncology nurses in both cities has been wonderful.

As someone with multiple myeloma, I will tell you that you need support from many places. I told my family and close friends. I told my dean and chairman of the department at my university. I soon decided that I would need the support of all my colleagues and told them. Then I announced it to my students in class. Their support came at different times, but it was always appreciated—none more so than a call I received from a friend who is a cardiologist on the first day of chemotherapy when I was feeling awful and was anxious about the whole thing. He provided just the right amount of information and more than the right amount friendship at a crucial time.

What's helped me get through this is not just support from people I love, but often from people I just met. We met an acupuncturist at a holiday party (before I knew definitively I had multiple myeloma) and decided that it was no accident that she was there that night. I've had an appointment with her almost every week during my journey and her treatments have lessened the feeling of being beaten up by the MM therapy. I went to see a counselor to help work with the many personal issues related to having a condition like multiple myeloma. The counseling took a lot of the emotional stress out of having a disease, particularly as I am from a family where we are expected to be strong.

My biggest challenges in dealing with multiple myeloma were that the early treatments made me feel worse. During the first month, I felt so badly I didn't know if I'd be able to continue with treatment. I had to really push through at that time, and it helped enormously knowing that the care I was getting was the best. I also had to overcome my anxiety of having lots of needles stuck in me!

But, what has been the most important thing for me has been to focus on having a life rather than a disease. Often, you'll find that online support groups are more focused on having an illness rather than having a life. When we have an appointment in Los Angeles with Dr. Berenson, we plan visits to museums, have meals at great places (often with Dr. B and his amazing wife Debra—both of whom we cherish), do a little shopping, and always go over to the ocean to receive some support from nature.

You also need to focus on a reason for living. My relationship with Susan has been important in my desire to get well. She also has provided the support and love that has helped me get well.

I would also suggest that you learn enough about the disease and its treatment so you have some idea of what's going on rather than just having stuff done to you. And absolutely seek out someone who specializes in multiple myeloma rather than relying on general oncologists, because they just can't know everything about every cancer. I've learned so much from Dr. Berenson about multiple myeloma and I appreciate him and his staff every day.

The experience of having cancer has been very different than I thought it would be. Of course, I thought I'd never have it. I also thought a cancer diagnosis meant a slow and painful death. It's been anything but that. After getting past the initial shock, having multiple myeloma made me examine my life from physical, emotional, spiritual, and mental perspectives. I appreciate more the people I love. I am grateful for the help I've received and the healing that has taken place and continues to take place.

Susan

When I first heard the words multiple myeloma, I couldn't believe it. I had lost both my parents to cancer, and I wasn't about to lose my husband. Fortunately, after many, many days of anxious moments, finally meeting with Dr. Berenson was a huge relief. We've never looked back from that day. We just went forward, confident that the best person on the earth was taking care of him. I remember leaving Dr. Berenson's office and saying to my husband, "Thank God, we have found our guy!" Steve has had such good response to treatment that each time we go to LA I feel even more grateful and lucky.

The initial shock of hearing that the person you love most in the world has cancer is devastating. I shook for at least three days. I got shingles. And until we knew how treatable multiple myeloma was, I had to think about what life would be without Steve. But after his first myeloma test numbers dropped significantly (a very good thing!), I knew eventually he would be well. That it was just a matter of time. That we were going to have a much, much longer time together. Wow. Other than being loved, it was the biggest gift I ever received.

I wouldn't have made it without my friends and family. At first, I was only going to tell a few people, but my best friend told me that, no, I was going to need a team of support for Steve and another one just for me. No wonder she's my best friend. As a support person for someone with cancer, you're going to need your own help. Be there always for whoever has cancer, but take time to take care of yourself. At first that seems impossible, but it gets easier as time goes by. Take a walk as often as possible. Go have lunch with friends. Laugh. Especially laugh. I would send email updates to people with Steve's progress so they would know how he was doing and, for some, what to continue to pray for. Find ways to release your own stress, even if it's a bath at the end of the day.

As shocking as it was, it's really been an amazing gift to think you're going to lose someone and then not lose them. It puts everything into focus. I don't worry about much or stress out over stupid things. I know what's important. It's love. Everything else is just stuff. Love.

I wish you the best of health in your journey and please know that there are amazing doctors, researchers, and mice working hard at the Institute for Myeloma & Bone Cancer Research (IMBCR) to rid the world of multiple myeloma. I know they'll do it.

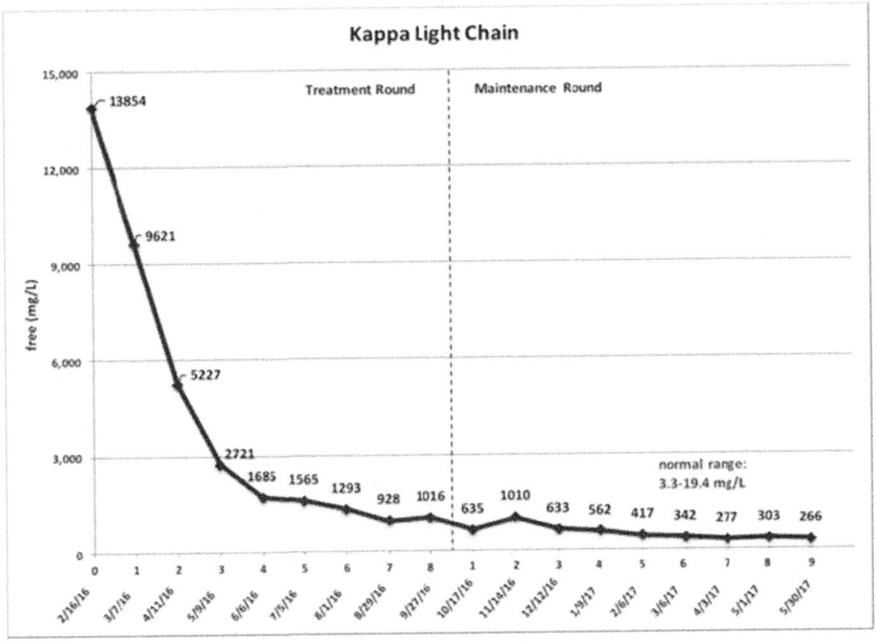

I Have WHAT???

By Susan K. -- MULTIPLIE MYELOMA?!!

Age: 60s

Teacher

Life is an interesting adventure. But, my definition of adventure was very different prior to 2010. I'm Susan, and this is my story. Ted, my husband, and I were comfy cozy in our fun world of traveling to international and domestic locales, essentially "winging it," focused on mixing in with the people wherever we were. Thoughts of future trips would swirl around immediately upon returning home. Is there a "Gypsy" gene?

Our other main focus was, and continues to be, serving as church counselors and counselor supervisors at Saddleback Church in Lake Forest, CA. That remains relatively unchanged as far as the time we serve.

At the end of the first decade of the 2000s, this adventure had a new face. And so it began with a diagnosis of breast cancer, followed by surgery, chemotherapy, and radiation. It's amazing how time came to a standstill for me, and how I seemed to zone out into that world of a multitude of emotions: shock, disbelief, denial, anxiety, and fear. As a retired teacher and a certified control freak, the loss of control was more than I could bear. Hadn't I done everything perfectly? A vigorous exercise program, an extremely healthy diet, a deep and abiding faith…what was going on?

Well, what was going on was the false assumption that I did indeed have it all under control. That lasted until I no longer had it all under control. And, so, I chose to embark on the very painful process of grieving my losses and working through these volatile emotions. To add insult to injury, the breast cancer chemotherapy threw me into a depression accompanied by a host of other feelings that were previously mentioned.

And, yes, I had multiple pity parties (nobody came), whining sessions, and lengthy crying periods. Ted looked like a deer in the headlights, totally unsure how to handle a wife who was all over the map. But, as all this played out, I was determined to maintain my current lifestyle as much as possible. Our ministry continued, and so did my running, which served to even me out. Social contacts were ongoing, as was gardening and traveling, but we scaled back to short trips. The motto: "Keep on keeping on."

Who was instrumental in helping me work through this mishmash? God, a loving and supportive husband, family, friends, staff and counselors at the church, and a great therapist, all for whom I am more than grateful for their compassionate prodding and gentle persuasion.

By the time the multiple myeloma diagnosis came down in 2011, I had worked through a lot of "baggage." But that remains, for me, an ongoing process. And, by the way, had it not been for the breast cancer, I'm not sure how far the myeloma would have progressed before it was discovered. I had a post treatment (breast) PET scan, which picked up the plasmacytoma, a mass of myeloma, on my sternum. Isn't life interesting?

So, how did I find Dr. Berenson? Over the years I had stayed in contact with a doctor who is now part of the National Institute of Health, in Baltimore, Maryland. Without hesitation, he strongly recommended that I see Dr. Berenson. It took one visit, and Ted and I knew, we just knew, we were firmly on board. His unique and uplifting style coupled with humor and a positive, caring attitude is absolutely delightful; which is not to take anything away from the fact that he's also cutting edge. Every single person on staff creates a warm and loving environment, an oasis.

Dr. Berenson brings to mind a quote from Jack Kemp, the politician and football great: "The power of one man or woman doing the right thing for the right reason, and at the right time, is the greatest influence in our society."

I Have WHAT???

By Susan N. -- MULTIPLE MYELOMA?!!

Age: 70s

Retired Social Worker

Twelve years ago, in 2003, I went to a neurosurgeon because I had excruciating pain that kept increasing. The doctor looked at the MRI and saw fractured vertebrae, which were pushing against my spinal cord. Within ten minutes, I was on a gurney and admitted to St. Vincent Hospital in Portland, Oregon. I was diagnosed with multiple myeloma.

The doctor knew that myeloma had weakened my bones. Since I could have become paralyzed without surgery, the doctor fused my thoracic spine.

While I was in rehab, I heard about the support group for myeloma patients sponsored by the Leukemia and Lymphoma Society (LLS). I asked the doctor if I could go to a meeting. I was wheeled to the group. I immediately realized I was not alone in navigating my myeloma journey.

During the 12 years that I have participated in the group, I have cried and laughed as each of us has told our stories. I felt the healing energy of support group members when I had a lumbar spine fusion and other medical procedures.

I went to Los Angeles to participate in a clinical trial conducted by Dr. James Berenson of the Institute for Myeloma and Bone Cancer Research. My T-cells were infused with a super active protein to make them work more effectively as they regenerate. My husband Phil continues to chant a mantra, "The T-cells. They stay active. They wrap their arms around the myeloma cells and usher them out."

Not all the myeloma cells can be "ushered out." Instead, they become "sleepy." I have had several chemotherapies that stabilize the myeloma. I have learned to "watch and wait." I start another treatment when the myeloma cells increase.

Phil and I had been married for eight years when I was diagnosed. I wanted to celebrate our 10th anniversary in Mendocino, my favorite place in northern California. I imagined we would walk along coastal trails that I had hiked many times before I had moved to Portland. Being able to hike meant I was becoming stronger despite yet another fractured vertebra. But instead of showing Phil the reconstructed village settled by Russians, I became sick with encephalitis, a brain infection. I couldn't visualize flying back to Portland on a crowded plane. We heard about a pilot who flew out of a small airport. When we talked to him, he offered to fly us at cost to Portland.

When I was diagnosed, a doctor told me to "get my affairs in order" because the survival rate was just a few years. Thanks to the new treatment options, multiple myeloma is becoming a chronic illness. Now I get an infusion once a month to keep my bones strong. No more burst vertebrae, hopefully!

While I was working as a social worker, I became interested in Viktor Frankl who wrote *Man's Searching for Meaning.* He wrote that we can choose our response to whatever happens in our lives. I have a dedicated oncologist and dedicated nurses rooting for all of their patients. The LLS has provided a support group that reminds me that I have the inner resources to live with myeloma until there is a cure.

I Have WHAT???

By Theresa F. -- MULTIPLE MYELOMA?!!

Age: 40s

Westlake Myeloma Support Group

Have you ever woken up and known that one day would change your entire life? My story began in late February 2008 with what I thought was a bad flu. I was having really bad migraines for days and knew something was wrong. The symptoms were getting worse, resulting in a high fever and the feeling that I was hearing people speak in the third person. I called my doctor finally knowing that this was not the flu. I was told to come in the next day and go to the ER if the fever got worse overnight.

The next day I went in for a chest X-ray and they discovered that I had double pneumonia and I was told to go immediately to the hospital to be admitted. Once in the ICU my kidneys began to slowly shut down. Because of the double pneumonia, my right lung collapsed and I was put on a ventilator machine. I also needed four units of blood. During this time the doctors were trying to figure out what mysterious disease was causing such serious problems in a 43-year-old, previously healthy woman. Then the moment came for me to reveal to my family what I had been told by the doctors—that I had multiple myeloma.

I was in the hospital for a total of 14 days and was told I was lucky to be alive. I thought to myself, "How did I get here?" One day I was fine and then 14 days later I did not even recognize my own body. I had lost 15 pounds in those 14 days and I looked like I had just come from a concentration camp. I guess in some ways you can say I was a survivor but didn't realize what my future would hold. Nobody had the heart to tell me that life with cancer—multiple myeloma—was now going to be my new path in life.

I went home to a new world surrounded only with one thing on my mind: surviving. Every day was a struggle because of the need to eat every 10 minutes from 6:00 a.m. to 11:00 p.m. in order to put the needed weight back on that I had lost. Then there were the trips to the doctor's office for my chemo twice a week for my new "cocktail" to keep me alive. I could not walk without a walker in the beginning and then graduated to walking with a cane. Eventually came the day when I could walk around the block by myself—what an accomplishment! Then there were the days of living with severe pain in each leg for 24 hours a day. I had developed neuropathy, which was extremely painful and has been described by some sufferers as frostbite-like discomfort. As I made it through each day, I wondered, *Why me? Why this new path?* I entered each stage from shock to anger to depression and finally to acceptance. The day finally came when the pain went away and life began again—my new path of "surviving."

I now have this new word in my vocabulary called *acceptance.* It took months to say the word or even think it, but I knew accepting was the only thing I could do, or multiple myeloma would consume me. I want to tell the world to be grateful for each day you have—you may not have another chance as I was given. My family and friends use the word *miracle* to describe my story, and I too know it was just that. I hope nobody has to say that "one day" changed their life. I am proud to say I just celebrated six months of surviving HELL and back.

This is what I wrote at six months…and now look at me four years later.

I got diagnosed when I was 43 years old and I am 47 years old now.

My family and friends had spent many hours researching when I was diagnosed, as many caregivers do when they hear such news. I had gone to City of Hope and UCLA for their thoughts and was told I needed a stem cell transplant.

I do think things happen for a reason—I had been turned down by my insurance for the stem cell transplant because they considered it experimental. So my third appointment was with Dr. Berenson and I know he saved my life.

I am no longer working—with myeloma, we never know how we'll feel. There are good days and then there are days that are harder. I have been very active with the Westlake Myeloma Support Group for the past four years, and it's been very rewarding for me. Funny that once we take the focus off of our own cancer, we can begin to start living again.

THE DOCTORS

AND

OTHER HEALTHCARE

PROFESSIONALS

You Have…

MULTIPLE MYELOMA!

WALDENSTROM'S MACROGLOBULINEMIA!

AMYLOIDOSIS!

MGUS!

(Monoclonal Gammopathy of Undetermined Significance)

By James R. Berenson, MD -- Oncologist

Medical and Scientific Director

Institute for Myeloma & Bone Cancer Research

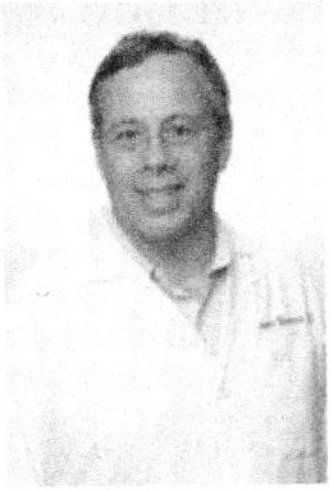

I am writing this to help patients who face multiple myeloma, Waldenstrom's macroglobulinemia, amyloidosis, or MGUS (monoclonal gammopathy of undetermined significance). I hope my thoughts will help all of you in your journey to make your life the very best while you are dealing with these disorders.

I think it is important to remember that we have made tremendous strides in just the past decade, with new drugs and treatment regimens that have greatly extended the lives of our patients and are also much better tolerated with fewer side effects. Ten years ago, treatments were not very effective, and the disease and regimens caused much suffering for our patients. Today, many of our patients live fully active lives while undergoing treatment. They climb Mount Kilimanjaro, hike the Great Wall of China, go on African safaris, mountain-bike in Colorado, and travel to all parts of the world. They work as lawyers, doctors, pharmacists, nurses, clergy, engineers, auto mechanics, truck drivers, movie directors, teachers, singers, actors, musicians, policemen, firemen, bankers, and builders. They enjoy their many hobbies—everything from running marathons, skiing, surfing, bike-riding, taking walks, gardening, baking a pie or batch of cookies for friends or fellow patients in clinic, playing the guitar, to simply reading a good book. They enjoy time with their children, grandchildren, great grandchildren, and their many friends. We expect that the next decade will bring us even more good news in terms of new therapies that will produce better quality lives for our patients facing these disorders.

What can you do to help your path with this disease, so that you can live your life to its fullest? Remember that you know yourself better than anyone! Be your own advocate. Don't be afraid to communicate how you feel to your healthcare professional. Tell him or her the good, the bad, and the ugly, not only regarding the disease's effects, but also the treatment's impact on your life. This may seem obvious, but I know that many of you fear that your doctor won't want to be bothered with this. Or, perhaps you feel that your doctor won't take the time to hear everything that is going on in your life as you face this disease. If your doctor resists, you need to speak up and say: "I matter as much as my disease." Don't be afraid to seek change in the captain of your ship if yours is not aboard in the way you need.

You should also tell your doctor if you aren't doing things as prescribed. In many cases, that may be fine, but your doctor should be in the know in case your changes cause problems that you are not aware of.

Don't be afraid to ask questions. I always say there is no question that is not worth asking if you think it is worth asking.

Don't be afraid to say, "I just don't get it." Many times, it is not you but your doctor who did not get it right or explain it clearly.

It's also quite okay to make suggestions to your physician on how you think things could be done better. That may pertain to a medication you are taking, a blood draw, the time you have to be in clinic, or even the temperature of the exam room.

I'm always grateful when patients bring new, potential treatments to my attention. Make sure that your doctor has an open mind and is willing to hear new approaches to your disorder—not only treatments for your disease but also ways to reduce the side effects from the treatments. I have learned a lot from listening to patients during my career. These little pearls have really changed lives for the better—not only for those of the patients providing the information, but many others, and it is thanks to many of our patients' own discoveries that the lives of so many have improved.

It is also important to remember that you are more than just a disease. The doctor's focus has to be on all of you. For example, many patients have plenty of bone problems from these diseases that their cancer doctors largely don't address; their focus is only on treating the cancer. Trained specialists can greatly improve these bone issues with minimal maneuvers. Similarly, nerve problems, whether issues with mental function or numbness and tingling, can significantly negatively impact quality of life, and many doctors do not adequately deal with these important issues. I always like to say, "Keep your eye on the ball, and the ball is the person, not the disease."

Remember that you are unique. You are not like any other patient. You have your own needs, wants, problems, families, friends, lifestyle, goals, and feelings that make you who you are. I like to quote what my wife's director, Geo Hartley, says when he directs actors: "It's not about more. It's about being more specific." We are working toward that with our new drugs, but that also means we need to work on that with each of you and treat you as the individual that you are.

I hope that each of you finds these words helpful in your journey with one of these disorders. Remember that with each year you are celebrating the victories that we, you and I, and many other researchers and doctors, have all helped bring to bear on these diseases. We all look forward to an amazing future for all of you.

FAQ 1: What Is Myeloma?

The first question patients ask us is: "What is this disease?" Multiple myeloma is a form of cancer that involves certain types of white blood cells found in the bone marrow. These cells are called plasma cells. Normally, they make up a small percentage of the bone marrow cells. Each plasma cell actually makes a single antibody. Even though they are present in small numbers, altogether the bone marrow plasma cells normally make many different types of antibodies that help fight infections. In multiple myeloma patients, there are too many plasma cells in the bone marrow that developed from a single abnormal cell. All of these clonal cells produce the same exact type of antibody as the original abnormal cell. These patients usually produce very little of the other types of antibodies to help fight infections, however.

FAQ 2: What Symptoms Are Associated with Multiple Myeloma?

The first thing patients want to know is how is this disease, multiple myeloma, going to affect me, and what kinds of problems might I encounter because of it? Multiple myeloma is a bone marrow-based cancer. Bone marrow is where blood cells are produced. This includes red blood cells, white blood cells, and platelets. When the weeds that are the plasma cells are malignant and take over the bone marrow, the green grass (normal bone marrow) can't grow. As a result, you are unable to grow red cells, white cells, and platelets. When you don't make red cells, you become anemic, and you could be tired and short of breath. When you don't make white cells, you don't have the ability to fight off infections. When you don't make platelets, you can have bleeding problems. Most commonly, myeloma reduces red blood cell production, and, thus, you become anemic.

Each healthy plasma cell makes one type of antibody. In myeloma, the malignant plasma cells are all of one type. Lots of this one protein is found in the blood. Unfortunately, certain types of these circulating antibodies can get through the filtering system in the kidneys and cause them to not function properly.

Because the bone marrow resides next to the bone, the myeloma-infested bone marrow often can wreak havoc on the bones. What does that mean? Bone loss, and when you lose bone, you fracture. You can also have bone pain from fractures and the direct expansion of the bone from the myeloma. Patients often present with fractures and bone pain. They also typically complain of height loss from fractures in the spine.

In addition, patients may have an increased number of infections because they make very little other antibodies except the monoclonal one. Without all of the normal antibodies, they have an impaired immune system. They also sometimes develop low white counts, which can make them susceptible to infections.

Myeloma is most often identified from routine blood tests. These may show either a low red blood cell count, i.e., anemia, or a high total protein level from all of the monoclonal antibody in their blood.

In terms of symptoms, back pain or bone pain is often present. You typically undergo X-ray evaluations in order to determine whether you have holes in the bones, so-called lytic lesions, or fractures. One of these findings may suggest that you have multiple myeloma. Other complaints may be fatigue or tiredness from low blood counts. The myeloma itself can cause these symptoms since they produce proteins that make you tired. You may also present with kidney failure. The symptoms of this condition include fatigue, nausea, vomiting, or the inability to have any urine output, which, in that case, means it is very severe. You may also experience frequent occurrence of infections prior to your diagnosis. This is due to a low white count, reduced normal antibody levels, and other problems with your immune system that result from your multiple myeloma.

Myeloma is a bone marrow based disease that can cause problems with your bones, kidneys, and immune system. Not just the bone marrow itself.

FAQ 3: How Is Multiple Myeloma Diagnosed?

How does the doctor actually make the diagnosis of myeloma or, in fact, rule it out? There are a series of tests and X-rays that are done in order to establish the diagnosis and determine the severity of the illness. First, we determine whether there is a monoclonal antibody, also called the M-protein, in the blood and urine. If present, we quantify the amount of it in the blood and in a 24-hour urine collection. Recently, a newer test called a "serum free light chain assay" is performed. It can measure a part of the monoclonal antibody in the blood. Together, these tests help establish whether the patient has an abnormal or monoclonal antibody. Measuring the amount of this protein helps determine whether it is at a level that is high enough to classify you as having myeloma or its premalignant version, monoclonal gammopathy of undetermined significance (MGUS). Blood tests are also done to determine whether you are anemic, if your kidneys are functioning properly, and whether your calcium level may be high. If the bone loss is severe, calcium levels can become very high in the blood and can cause serious medical problems.

A bone marrow examination is performed. Both a small amount of liquid bone marrow and a solid piece are removed from the lower back or upper hip, the iliac bone in the lower back. This determines whether abnormal plasma cells are present and the percentage of them and helps determine whether the patient has MGUS or multiple myeloma. In addition, further testing is done on the bone marrow to determine whether the abnormal plasma cells show chromosomal or genetic abnormalities. The results of these tests can help determine the relative severity of the disease and can be helpful in making decisions about how much and what type of treatment is necessary.

And last but not least, X-rays are done of the bones to determine whether holes are present. These are also known as lytic lesions, and they result from excessive bone loss in specific anatomic sites. In addition, the X-rays may show fractures. Sometimes additional imaging is done through MRIs, CT or PET CT scans. These more precisely identify lesions and to determine whether those holes or lesions in the bones may lead to problems that may require surgical intervention or radiation therapy, and, in some cases, help to classify if patients require treatment or not for their monoclonal gammopathy condition.

FAQ 4: How Do You Know If You Need Treatment?

So, the next question the myeloma patient has is, "Do I need treatment?" Many patients with myeloma need very little treatment, since this disease can progress very slowly. Sometimes, the patient's myeloma initially requires no treatment. In some cases, they may never require therapy. Importantly, we continue to discover new drugs that will hopefully benefit you when you need them. Your doctor has to be careful not to over-treat your disease. The decision to treat is the first one.

It turns out that most individuals with a monoclonal antibody or M-protein in their blood and/or urine don't have myeloma. They, in fact, have a disorder called MGUS, or monoclonal gammopathy of an undetermined significance, in which the amount of abnormal protein is lower (see section of book regarding MGUS for more details). They also don't have evidence of low blood counts or anemia. They don't have significant bone disease, high calcium, or kidney disease. Also, their bone marrow shows very few plasma cells (less than 10%). Those patients can generally just be watched with periodic lab tests done every 6 months, although if they have evidence of bone loss such as osteopenia or osteoporosis they may require treatment with drugs to strengthen their bone like bisphosphonates which are administered intravenously when they come in for their lab tests.

Next, there is a group of patients who have what we call smoldering myeloma. This group represents about 10–15% percent of myeloma patients. They meet the diagnostic criteria for myeloma in that they have more than 10% plasma cells in their bone marrow. They do have myeloma but they don't have any clinical manifestations of the disease to make it necessary for them to need treatment. They don't have high calcium levels in the blood, kidney failure, low red blood cell count, or anemia. They don't have fractures or lots of holes in their bones. They don't feel poorly from what may be the myeloma. In fact, they're living a pretty normal life. Those patients generally may benefit simply from treatment with bone strengtheners like bisphosphonates if they have bone loss and may not require any other therapy. However, over time they can develop disease that requires treatment, especially if they become anemic, develop bone lesions, exhibit high calcium levels, or experience kidney failure related to their myeloma. Patients with smoldering myeloma can be classified into risk categories for developing disease that is more likely to require treatment sooner based on the percentage of plasma cells in the bone marrow, the size of the M-protein, whether they are able to still make normal antibodies, the levels of the serum free light chain, and the number of lesions on MRI. Recently, some of these patients with the high-risk features that indicate a higher likelihood of more quickly progressing to active myeloma have been reclassified as requiring immediate treatment. Specifically, those with a higher percentage of bone marrow plasma cells, increased serum free light chain levels, and more than one abnormality on their MRI are now considered to require immediate treatment. However, it remains unclear whether this early intervention improves their long-term outcome.

However, most patients with myeloma come in with one of the signs or symptoms that show that they need treatment. They feel poorly, and they may have bone pain associated with a fracture or holes in the bones. They may be weak and tired. They may have kidney failure and low blood counts, especially anemia, which also makes them feel weak and tired. Their blood calcium levels may be elevated from bone loss. Those patients require immediate treatment. That treatment can take on many variations, depending on the patient's specific type of myeloma as well as their other medical problems, and also their work and lifestyle.

FAQ 5: How Does Your Doctor Decide What the Right Treatment Is for You?

So now that the doctor has decided that you need treatment for your multiple myeloma, how do they decide what treatment should be given? That specific treatment will be based on several things. One factor that is very important, of course, is the collective characteristics of the disease. For example, is the bone marrow very involved with a lot of plasma cells, resulting in anemia or other low blood counts? Are there cells in the blood that are of the myeloma type? When these plasma cells are in the blood and have traveled outside of the bone marrow, which is known as plasma cell leukemia, it is a very serious form of myeloma. This is also the case if the myeloma has moved into other organs like the liver or pancreas. How involved are the bones? Are there just a few holes in the head? Are there lots of lesions all over the skeleton? Does the patient have bone pain as well as fractures from the bone loss? What are the genetic abnormalities in the cancer cells? They may suggest this is a poor risk patient that may require more aggressive treatment. What is the kidney function like? What is your lifestyle and work style? Are you a very active person? Are you running marathons, or are you bedridden from the effects of myeloma and were very active just a few months ago? We also want to know what your other medical conditions are. Maybe you already have kidney disease from diabetes or high blood pressure. Maybe you have heart failure. Are you able to take oral drugs correctly either by yourself or with supervision from a caregiver? These can impact the choices that the doctor will make to treat your multiple myeloma. For the patient who has been previously treated, you also want to know what specific treatments they have received before. How well did they work? How did they tolerate it? Did it cause side effects? Did they feel poorly on it? Were they nauseated? Did they have to stay at home because they were so tired from the treatment? Was it lowering their blood counts, which caused delays in further treatment? Was it affecting their liver and kidney function? All of these should be considered in terms of what the doctors decide to treat you with. Treatment choices have become more complicated, thanks to the great increase in therapeutic options available today compared to just a few years ago when the choices were so limited.

FAQ 6: What Are the Treatment Options for Multiple Myeloma?

So, what are the treatment options today for myeloma patients? Well, there are so many more ways to treat this disease than just a few years ago. The general classes of drugs used to treat myeloma included only chemotherapy along with steroids. More recently, we have the immunomodulatory drugs thalidomide, followed by Revlimid, also known as lenalidomide, and now Pomalyst, also known as pomalidomide. We also have available three drugs with similar mechanisms of action; these are called "proteasome inhibitors." First, we had Velcade, also known as bortezomib, starting in the early 2000s. A second drug in this class has been used called Kyprolis, also known as carfilzomib. More recently, a pill version called Ninlaro, also known as ixazomib, became available.

Recently, two antibodies have been approved to treat multiple myeloma, Darzalex, also known as daratumumab, and Empliciti, also known as elotuzumab. These are the first antibody-based treatments available to treat this disease. These treatments target proteins present on myeloma tumor cells but also offer immune boosting effects that help make them work better.

In addition, a new class of drugs known as "histone deacetylase inhibitors" has shown benefits for treating myeloma patients. Recently, a drug with this activity, Farydak, also known as panobinostat, has become available to treat myeloma patients.

We also have drugs that are not approved for myeloma but can be used, such as arsenic trioxide, which is approved for a rare form of acute leukemia. In addition, there are lots of drugs now in development, including other antibodies and other targets that we will discuss in more detail as we address specific drug classes and options.

A key point we've learned over the last few years is that just because you're actually progressing or not being responsive to one drug does not mean that the same drug will not work when combined with another agent that has demonstrated benefit for myeloma patients. We've learned that with the proteasome inhibitors. For example, if Velcade was used and failed to work with a drug like Cytoxan, then the patient may respond when Velcade is combined with other drugs known to be active for myeloma, such as Doxil or steroids. The same is also true with immunomodulatory agents like thalidomide or Revlimid. What we have learned more recently is that even drugs in the same class that the patient has failed to respond to can produce responses when another drug from the same class is used. For example, patients who do not respond to Velcade when it is combined with the alkylating agent Cytoxan may respond to Velcade when it is combined with another alkylating agent called bendamustine. Even more startling, patients might be failing with one immunomodulatory agent, such as Revlimid in combination, but they may show responses when the same combination is used with another immunomodulatory agent such as Pomalyst or thalidomide. Similarly, we have shown that patients failing to respond to the proteasome inhibitor Velcade can often respond to the same combination when Velcade is replaced with another drug in the same class, which is Kyprolis, also known as carfilzomib.

Thus, the number of choices for myeloma patients today is so much greater. In the past, it was thought that myeloma patients showed class resistance, so that patients failing drugs in the same class would be unlikely to respond when another drug in the same class was tried. Clearly, this is not the case, as is demonstrated in many recently completed clinical studies.

FAQ 7: What Are the Specific Classes of Drugs Used to Treat Multiple Myeloma?

Let's Start with Chemotherapy

The oldest agents to treat myeloma are the chemotherapy drugs. Specific drug classes are effective in myeloma, especially the alkylating agents and anthracyclines.

The oldest drugs are the alkylating agents, including melphalan, cyclophosphamide, and most recently bendamustine. These drugs are not particularly active alone, but when used in combination with some other agents, which we will describe below, are very active. Drugs that are commonly used with alkylating agents include steroids, immunomodulatory agents, and the proteasome inhibitors. These drugs, when used at lower doses, have very few side effects and infrequently lower blood counts, but other than that and occasional nausea are very well tolerated when given for a few days every month. They can be quite effective for a long period of time. However, only when combined with other agents and classes of drugs used to treat myeloma today do they produce significant clinical benefits for myeloma patients.

Drugs in the other major chemotherapy class used to treat myeloma today are the anthracyclines. The oldest agent was doxorubicin or Adriamycin, but in the last few years a newer and safer version has been developed called Doxil or Lipodox, also known as pegylated liposomal doxorubicin, which is a chemically modified form of doxorubicin. It's like having the drug in a fat globule. It can be given very safely and is very active to treat myeloma patients. When given alone, it does not have much clinical activity, but when combined with steroids and especially proteasome inhibitors such as Velcade or Kyprolis it's quite active. Also, the same is true when these drugs are given with immunomodulatory agents, especially Revlimid and more recently Pomalyst.

When Doxil or Lipodox are given conventionally once every three weeks, they can cause significant side effects such as mucositis, so that the inside of the mouth can hurt, and a skin condition called hand-foot syndrome, which is associated with blistering and red, hot hands and feet, especially on the palms and the soles. This can be quite troubling for patients. We now know that these side effects can be greatly reduced and pretty much eliminated when we simply give Doxil at lower doses more often—twice weekly rather than a higher dose once every three weeks. The other side effect that may occur long-term with anthracyclines is heart failure. However, this occurs only after several years of usage, and long-term usage of these drugs for myeloma patients is uncommon. In addition, the newer forms, Doxil and Lipodox, are safer, so heart failure is very rarely a problem anymore with drugs in this class. Regardless, it remains important for patients to have their heart function checked with heart tests such as an echocardiogram or MUGA scan to assure that it is adequate before they initiate treatment with Doxil, Lipodox, or Adriamycin.

FAQ 8: Why Are Steroids Used to Treat Myeloma and Which Ones Are Used?

One of the most active drugs to treat myeloma today is a steroid. These are not the same steroids that athletes have used; these are the steroids that, in fact, are commonly used to calm down inflammation. These are called glucocorticosteroids. They are also known as corticosteroids, and include drugs such as prednisone, methylprednisolone or Medrol, and dexamethasone or Decadron. These can be given orally or intravenously to treat myeloma patients. We know that the steroids directly can kill the myeloma cells, but, equally important, they can make the soil less hospitable for the myeloma to grow in, if you will. It's no longer fertile, it's barren soil, and the myeloma dies and the patient feels better. Steroids remain an excellent drug choice for myeloma patients today. They can be very easily and effectively combined with all of the other active drugs used to treat myeloma, such as chemotherapy agents, proteasome inhibitors, and immunomodulatory agents. They are, in fact, among the most active drugs to treat myeloma and they are certainly by far the cheapest. The problem is that their dosing and schedules can have a major impact on their tolerability, and even different ones can have marked differences in potency and side effects. Patients may also develop cataracts after long-term use.

Some patients don't like being on steroids. However, it turns out the dose, specific steroid, and dosing schedule are very important in determining the patient's ability to stay on these drugs with minimal negative effects. In our own practice, we believe that intravenous treatment results in fewer side effects, less inability to sleep (so-called insomnia), less hyperactivity, and reduced negative effects on mood. We also believe that when given as a pill, methylprednisolone or Medrol appears to be better tolerated, especially when given at lower doses every other day, than the other steroid drugs such as dexamethasone or prednisone.

Studies done recently have shown that the amount of steroids that we used up until recently was much too much. These led to poor outcomes for patients because of the many side effects that patients experienced. Problems when taking the drugs at the higher doses included more infections, blood clots, and increased blood sugar. The results of a recent randomized trial showed us that less was, in fact, "more," as patients were able to remain on their treatment, resulting in improved outcomes with reduced doses of steroids. With lower doses and differences in types and routes of administration, patients are able to live happier and more fulfilling lives while taking these drugs.

Even if these are older drugs, steroids really do work, especially when used in combination with other medications, and they can, in fact, have the added benefit of reducing side effects associated with other drugs. We have also learned that when you combine these drugs with other anti-myeloma drugs, you can effectively administer lower amounts of the steroids. This results in far fewer side effects than we used to observe before we had the opportunity to combine these drugs with all of the new types of drugs to treat myeloma patients.

FAQ 9: What Is the Role of Proteasome Inhibitors for Treating Myeloma?

Another class of drugs commonly used to treat myeloma today is the proteasome inhibitors. This started with bortezomib or Velcade more than a decade ago. These drugs, in fact, enable other drugs to knock out myeloma much better. We call these drugs "chemosensitizers." They make the other drugs, such as the chemotherapy drugs and steroids, work much better to eliminate the myeloma tumor cells. We know they can directly kill myeloma, as well as also make myeloma cells unable to grow. They have a multitude of different ways in which they accomplish these goals, but basically they inhibit a system in our cells that is like a garbage can and gets rid of all the toxic stuff. When the garbage can is closed with a proteasome inhibitor, toxic proteins accumulate and they cause myeloma cells to die. The good news is that myeloma cells are much more sensitive to this impact than other healthy cells in the body.

Velcade was first used to treat late-stage myeloma, but today is often given as front-line treatment for myeloma. Its activity is much better when it is combined with steroids, chemotherapy, and immunomodulatory agents. Today, it is uncommon for Velcade to be used alone. These drugs can cause side effects, specifically and most commonly peripheral neuropathy with numbness and tingling, burning pain in the hands and feet, and sometimes weakness in the legs and the arms. These effects can be reduced if Velcade is given at lower doses, given in longer cycles, and if the drug is given subcutaneously instead of intravenously. These three things result in much less frequent occurrence and reduced severity of neuropathy. As a result, patients stay on drugs. Importantly, we've learned that when the drugs are combined together at these lower doses and for longer cycles, they can be very effective with markedly less side effects. Velcade can cause shingles, a type of viral infection that affects the skin, so we recommend that patients on this drug be treated with anti-viral drugs like Zovirax, also known as acyclovir, Valtrex, or Famvir while receiving them. If they're treated with Velcade, the drugs can also lead to reductions in blood counts, so we monitor those as well when patients are on this treatment. These are highly effective drugs that certainly improve the quality and the length of myeloma patients' lives today.

Another proteasome inhibitor called Kyprolis, or carfilzomib, was approved to treat myeloma patients in 2012. Although it is in the same drug class as Velcade and has similar mechanisms of actions, it turns out it can overcome resistance to Velcade in myeloma patients. Therefore, it is a great option for patients who have failed Velcade, as well as other immunomodulatory agents. It causes less neuropathy than Velcade and, therefore, is a good option for patients who have Velcade-induced neuropathy. Like Velcade, it is much more effective when combined with steroids, chemotherapy, or the immunomodulatory agents such as thalidomide, Revlimid, or

Pomalyst. Recent studies suggest that doses of the drug can be increased safely and suggest that it may be more effective than Velcade when both drugs are given with steroids. Rarely, it can cause heart problems, especially during the first few months of its administration. Thus, it is important to communicate to your health care professional team any possible heart-related symptoms such as chest pain, cough, shortness of breath, or fluid retention. Its schedule being on two consecutive days intravenously on a weekly basis can be quite inconvenient but recent studies show that once-weekly dosing at higher doses is also effective and safe.

In 2015, the first orally administered proteasome inhibitor became available. This drug, Ninlaro, also known as ixazomib, is taken once weekly on days 1, 8, and 15 of a four-week cycle. Its effectiveness appears to be similar to Velcade but it appears to cause less peripheral neuropathy. Similar to both Velcade and Kyprolis, it is much more active when combined with other drugs such as steroids, chemotherapy, and proteasome inhibitors. The advantage of an orally administered proteasome inhibitor may improve the ability of patients to remain on a proteasome inhibitor more long-term than the other two agents, Velcade and Kyprolis, which must be given in a clinic either intravenously or subcutaneously.

FAQ 10: What Are Immunomodulatory Agents and How Are They Used to Treat Myeloma?

Another class of drugs that's quite effective is the immunomodulatory agents. These included first Thalomid, also known as thalidomide, more recently Revlimid or lenalidomide, and even most recently Pomalyst or pomalidomide. These drugs are called immunomodulatory agents because they help boost the immune system and take away the part of the immune system that suppresses the immune functions from killing myeloma. They have many other ways that these drugs may eliminate the myeloma. They reduce blood vessels that feed the myeloma. They can also knock out the myeloma directly, and make the neighborhood in which the myeloma cells grow less hospitable for that to happen. These drugs are not only active as single agents but their activity is greatly boosted when combined with other drugs such as steroids, chemotherapy, or the proteasome inhibitors, such as Velcade or Kyprolis. The other good news is that when they are combined, their doses can be reduced, and, therefore, they cause fewer side effects.

The problems with thalidomide specifically are peripheral neuropathy, which manifests itself as numbness, tingling, and sometimes burning pain, and is usually irreversible. All three drugs can also cause constipation, and certainly can increase the risk of blood clots in the legs and lungs, especially when combined with steroids and some specific types of chemotherapy. The drugs are very active and can be given for a long period of time, but there seems to be a small risk of secondary cancers, especially lymphoma and leukemia, that has been recognized recently with long-term use of Revlimid. Their ability to improve survival in myeloma patients far outstrips their very low risk of causing a secondary cancer. The risk of these secondary malignancies seems to be especially increased among patients taking Revlimid who have been treated with high-dose chemotherapy, specifically melphalan, followed by transplantation of stem cells. Side effects of these drugs may also include tiredness, as well as inability to think clearly. But lowering the dose can certainly help overcome these problems. When these drugs are given in the evening, it also reduces this side effect as well. Since the drugs are cleared in the kidney, patients may require a reduction in the dose. We know that's true for Revlimid, but not so true for thalidomide, and appears not to be required for patients taking Pomalyst either. However, all three of these drugs certainly can be given safely to patients with poor renal function or kidney function. You just have to reduce the dose if the patient is taking Revlimid. In terms of reducing the clot risk, we simply have a patient take baby aspirin in order to help prevent this complication. Some patients may require stronger drugs such as warfarin, also known as Coumadin, to prevent clots, especially patients that are overweight, diabetic, or have a prior history of a clotting event.

These are a very active class of drugs, especially when combined with chemotherapy drugs, steroids, or the proteasome inhibitors.

FAQ 11: What Is a Histone Deacetylase Inhibitor and How Is it Useful to Treat Myeloma?

Histones are proteins that cover the DNA in the nucleus. These proteins regulate expression of genes. These proteins' ability to regulate gene expression is controlled through chemical structures that are present on them known as acetylated forms. When they are present, gene expression is upregulated and when they are reduced, gene expression is reduced. It turns out that in cancer cells there are too little of these acetylated forms present on histones because of increased activity of the type of proteins called histone deacetylases, which remove the acetylated forms, and underactivity of the proteins called histone acetylases, which place these structures on the histones. The net result is, with too little of the acetylated forms on histones, there is reduced expression of genes, especially of genes that lead to the production of proteins that turn off cancer growth. Thus, reversing this process by increasing these acetylated forms on histones should increase expression of genes and result in higher levels of proteins that turn off cancer growth. To accomplish this, inhibitors of the histone deacetylase have been developed, resulting in approval of several drugs that block this protein for treating a variety of cancers related to myeloma. In myeloma, these drugs are specifically thought to enhance the effectiveness of proteasome inhibitors by also leading to the accumulation of toxic, misfolded proteins in tumor cells beyond what the proteasome inhibitors do alone. Recently, a drug in this class has been specifically approved for treating myeloma, Farydak, or panobinostat. Although this drug shows very little effectiveness when administered alone, it improves the activity of steroids and Velcade when the three drugs are combined together compared to the latter two agents without

Farydak, possibly due to its increasing levels of misfolded proteins within the myeloma tumor cells as mentioned above. The drug shows significant side effects, however. Fatigue, gastrointestinal problems, and low blood counts commonly occur among patients receiving Farydak and are increased when the drug is used in combination with Velcade.

FAQ 12: How Do Antibodies Work to Treat Multiple Myeloma?

Antibodies are proteins that specifically bind to target proteins. In myeloma, two antibodies have been developed that target proteins that are preferentially present on the tumor cells in myeloma patients. In addition, recent studies show that these antibodies also enhance the immune system's ability to eliminate the tumor cells.

Specifically, Empliciti, or elotuzumab, binds to a protein called "signaling lymphocyte activation molecule factor 7," also known as SLAMF7, that is present on myeloma tumor cells and natural killer cells, a type of cell that is involved in the immune system's ability to eliminate cancer cells. In myeloma patients, Empliciti binds to the myeloma tumor cell, setting it up for elimination. When Empliciti binds to the immune natural killer cells, it paradoxically stimulates their immune activity because these cells contain specific factors not present on myeloma cells. These factors not only protect the natural killer cell from being eliminated by the antibody binding to their SLAMF7 but actually stimulate them to function as "eliminators" of the myeloma cells that are bound with antibody to the same target protein, SLAMF7. Thus, this combination of enhancement of natural killer cell immune activity with targeting of the tumor cell by Empliciti leads to myeloma cell death. In clinical trials, the drug does not show activity unless it is combined with Revlimid and steroids. It improves upon the activity of Revlimid and steroids in myeloma patients and this led to the approval for this drug in late 2015 to treat previously treated myeloma patients with this three-drug combination. It is well tolerated but must be administered intravenously once weekly for several months before patients change to an every-other-week schedule.

CD38 is present at high levels on myeloma tumor cells. Antibodies to CD38 have been developed to treat myeloma patients. In late 2015, Darzalex, also known as daratumumab, was approved when administered alone to treat myeloma patients based on a trial showing modest activity in previously treated patients. It has significant allergic-type infusion reactions, especially during the first time it is administered, occasionally leading to permanent discontinuation of the drug in some patients. However, after the first several doses these reactions only rarely occur. Because of the drug-related infusion reactions, the drug is administered intravenously over many hours the first time a patient undergoes treatment but this is shortened during subsequent infusions during the first month of weekly administration. The drug is then given every other week for several months followed by ongoing monthly administration. The drug can also complicate blood banking procedures to match blood for a certain blood type. Importantly, the activity of steroids with either Velcade or Revlimid is greatly improved when Darzalex is added into the regimen. In addition, the combination of this antibody treatment with Pomalyst and steroids has been shown to be effective and is now approved for use to treat MM patients who have failed other therapies.

Other antibodies are also in development targeting similar proteins as well as novel ones. In addition, studies are beginning to combine the targeting power of these types of antibodies for the cancer cell with toxins that are attached to the antibody, allowing high concentrations of the toxin to specifically be delivered to the tumor cell and sparing the rest of the body of untoward effects from the toxin.

FAQ 13: How Is Arsenic Trioxide Useful for Treating Multiple Myeloma?

Now that you've heard about five recently approved new drugs to treat myeloma—Revlimid, thalidomide, Pomalyst, Velcade, and Kyprolis—let's talk about another relatively new drug that's approved to treat leukemia APL, but not myeloma, arsenic trioxide. This is a heavy metal that is showing great efficacy for treating myeloma patients today, especially when used in combination therapies. We don't completely understand how it works, but we do know that, like Velcade, it also prevents the breakdown of proteins that cause myeloma cells to die. It also potently inhibits the formation of blood vessels that we know are also important in the growth of myeloma. The drug is administered intravenously. It usually takes several hours to administer it. It's given a couple of times weekly, although the schedules vary. It has a distinctly separate side-effect profile; specifically, the drug can slow the heart rate, and so we monitor the electrocardiogram or EKG periodically for patients who are receiving it. EKGs are monitored weekly, and then monthly after the first several months. It's rare that heart rhythm changes occur, but it can be serious if this happens. Importantly, to reduce this side effect, we have to keep the potassium and magnesium levels on the higher side of the normal range, which reduces the risk. Rarely, this drug can cause numbness or tingling in the hands and feet. Importantly, Vitamin C increases the effectiveness of arsenic trioxide by increasing free radicals in the myeloma cell. It's also been effective when combined with steroids and a variety of chemotherapy agents, and more recently thalidomide and Velcade.

FAQ 14: How Do Doctors Know If Your Treatment Is Working?

So how do we know if the treatment is working or not working? Well, we measure not the amount of tumor cells themselves that are in the bone marrow (you can't get to them), but their product, the antibody marker. Does it go up, stay the same, or go down? We measure that in the blood and the urine, and most patients have it in their blood. Sometimes about 15% of patients only have the protein in the urine; it's just a part of the antibody. We now have a newer assay, the serum free light chain, so we can perform that measurement of this light chain not only in the urine but also in the blood as well. When we measure the percentage change in the antibody protein marker from the level it was when you started treatment, we are able to determine the extent of your response. If it's 25–49% below where you started, it's called a minimal response or MR. 50–89% is partial response or PR, and at least 90%, but not completely gone, is a very good partial response or VGPR. If that marker disappears completely, we call it a complete response or CR. Changes in the amount of urine protein are also used to assess response but the percentage changes required for responses are different: at least 50% for an MR, more than 90% for PR.

These days it's fairly common for patients to respond to some degree, and many patients achieve complete responses. However, the achievement of complete response in which that protein marker disappears doesn't mean the patient is cured. It certainly can come back in time. When the protein marker reappears, we tell the patient, "Your disease is progressing." If it goes up by more than 25%, we also say you're progressing. We also want to know how you are tolerating the therapy. Are you feeling poorly? Are you tired? Are you having pain? Are you nauseated? That may make us want to change therapy, or at least reduce the dose. How it's impacting your blood counts or your kidney function also may lead to changes in the dose, or in the scheduling of the drugs. So, it's not necessarily all about whether the disease is getting worse or better, but also what the treatment is doing to your body and how you're feeling on it. Reductions in doses and changes in schedule of the drugs can often reduce any side effects and greatly improve their tolerability. Notably, today there are many other options that you can try if you are not tolerating your current therapy very well.

FAQ 15: How Long Do You Need to Stay on Treatment?

So, if I'm being treated, how long do I have to stay on the treatment? The data is emerging that maintaining the remission maintenance therapy is a key part of the treatment plan for your myeloma today. Early studies we and others performed first showed that steroids were effective, and more recent studies with Revlimid have shown an improvement in survival with their long-term use, although we certainly use the proteasome inhibitors, first Velcade and now Kyprolis, long term, and they seem to be very safe. There's really not a lot of randomized data that shows they are effective as maintenance agents, but we are also maintaining treatment with these drugs. We believe that patients need to stay on treatment because this disease remains incurable for the most part today, and we want you to stay in remission for as long as possible. We also, though, use lower doses and we give patients less of those drugs per month. This allows patients to come to the clinic less often to receive those drugs that require administration at the practice, such as the proteasome inhibitors Velcade or Kyprolis. However, giving drugs less often doesn't have to be the case if you are taking oral agents such as Revlimid and steroids. Maintaining the remission is a key part of the treatment plan. So, we do keep patients on treatment, but we often give the drugs at lower doses and less often. We try to make the schedules more convenient, and we certainly want patients to maintain their quality of life or to improve it when they move to the maintenance phase of their treatment. We discontinue the chemotherapy agents, such as Adriamycin, Doxil, cyclophosphamide, melphalan, and bendamustine, during the maintenance therapy because we know long term these drugs can cause permanent damage to the bone marrow. This may in the long term prevent the patient from receiving these and other drugs in new combination treatments.

FAQ 16: What Are Some of The New Agents in Development?

So, what's happening in myeloma today in terms of new agents? It's an explosion today. There are many new agents in development. The major agents in development that are most promising are newer antibodies and the antibody conjugates. We've used antibodies to treat other cancers very effectively, such as the lymphomas, the skin cancer melanoma, and some types of chronic leukemia, and until recently we did not have similar drugs approved to treat myeloma. However, there are now two approved antibodies recently approved to treat myeloma, Empliciti and Darzalex, and many more in development targeting the same proteins that these do, as well as other proteins.

The most exciting development during the last few years is the ability to combine these targeted antibodies with anti-myeloma drugs. So how does that help things? Because if we can deliver the drug just to the cancer cell, allowing the antibody to bind the cancer cell with the drug, then that drug can just get into the cancer cell. We can then deliver therapy that truly is tumor-specific and get much more of the drug inside the myeloma tumor cell, killing it and leaving the rest of the patient alone. And we're finally doing that in the laboratory, and actually curing mice with myeloma for the first time. We hope for that to happen in the clinic soon. Clinical trials are beginning to use this approach in myeloma patients. Some of these drugs are effectively now being used to treat other types of similar cancers, such as lymphomas.

Other promising studies are targeting other parts of the immune system. Recent studies suggest that drugs known as checkpoint inhibitors, which prevent functioning of proteins that block the immune response known as PD-1 and PDL-1 inhibitors, may be effective for treating myeloma patients, especially when combined with other drugs that are effective to treat myeloma patients. Checkpoint inhibitors have shown effectiveness to treat many other types of cancer in the past few years. In addition, manipulation of a type of immune cell called a T-lymphocyte to carry proteins that target myeloma cells appears promising from early trial results, but problems with serious side effects need to be controlled before this gains widespread usage.

We and others are also developing other drugs for myeloma patients that target the pathways within the cells that make myeloma tumor cells grow and prevent them from dying. These include the PI3 kinase inhibitors and many other targets in the myeloma cell.

In general, we hope over the next few years we are able to use drugs that will only attack the myeloma cell and leave the rest of the body alone. That's our goal now: to get therapy that truly is only tumor-specific.

FAQ 17: What Is Clinical Research and How Is It Carried Out?

You may be asked to participate in clinical research, and you may want to know what it is before you even decide that you want to participate. Clinical research involves the testing of drugs that we hope will help many patients, like you, with myeloma. In fact, there are many different types of clinical trials to determine whether drugs either are safe or more effective than the presently available agents. The clinical trials are done in stages ranging from Phase 1 to 4. In Phase 1 trials, we don't even know if the drug is safe. We are just trying to evaluate safety, but we may get a hint as to whether it has clinical activity. In Phase 2 trials, now that we know the proper dose that is safe and well-tolerated, we test it for patients with your disease. Once we establish that the drug has activity to knock out the myeloma, we move it into Phase 3 trials, in which we select some patients to receive the tried-and-true gold standard dose of the new treatment, which we hope is better. And finally, in Phase 4 trials, now that we know (ideally) the new treatment is better than the previous gold standard, it will be evaluated for other types of cancer patients or subsets of myeloma patients to further determine its effectiveness and safety. In addition, there may be slight tweaks with the treatment in terms of the regimen, how often we give it, or for how long, which may make it a more effective and safer drug for our patients.

There also may be trials that are called PK or PC trials. So, what are these? These are pharmacokinetic or pharmacodynamic trials. They do not necessarily test whether the drugs work, but correlate the drug levels and their biological effects with their clinical activity, and also determine other measures of outcome besides just the change in the patient's myeloma.

All of these trials help us in a way so that we can find the best ways to benefit many other patients like you. So, for you to make a decision about whether you want to participate in trials, you have to decide if the extra effort on your part is worth it. You may need to come to the clinic more often for additional blood draws and other tests that are part of the trial. You have to weigh that against the possible benefit for yourself and the many other patients like yourself that you will be helping over the long run.

Overall, clinical trials are a great thing to participate in because the old treatments from a few years ago, you have to remember, were once the new study treatments. The new treatments that we're testing in the clinic today will hopefully become the standard treatments a few years from now. All of these new drugs have helped lead to not only improvement in the length of lives for patients with myeloma, but just as important, benefitted their quality of life, as well.

FAQ 18: What Problems Might Arise in My Body from Having Multiple Myeloma?

Now that you've learned about all of the specific drugs to treat myeloma, over the next few sections we are going to tell you about the specific complications that occur in myeloma patients. You will find out how you can prevent them from occurring or at the very least reduce their impact on your life. These problems may arise from the disease itself or often from the treatments that are administered to treat the myeloma. In sections of the book written by specific healthcare professional experts, you will also find more information regarding many complications of the disease and how to prevent and treat them.

Bone Disease

The most important and common problems for myeloma patients are bone-related complications. Patients with myeloma lose bone. Why? Because the "Pac-Man" cell in the bone called the osteoclast is stimulated to actually get rid of bone by the myeloma cell. So, our job is to stop that osteoclast from activating and destroying bone. Fortunately, today we have drugs that help with this called bisphosphonates, which come in the form of a monthly infusion of either Zometa or Aredia. They have been shown to dramatically reduce the occurrence of fractures and spinal cord compression. Prior to bisphosphonates, patients often required radiation therapy or surgery, but these treatments are much less often required nowadays.

Keep in mind that bisphosphonates are very potent, and, as a result, can have a negative impact on the kidney. Thus, it's important that patients have monthly monitoring of their kidney function. Infrequently, patients also may have jaw problems known as osteonecrosis of the jaw, or ONJ, usually resulting from surgical procedures such as the extraction of teeth. So, maintaining dental health is a key to not only making sure these drugs are effective, but to reducing the risk of jaw problems that can frequently result from treatment with these drugs over the long term. About one-third of patients will develop flu-like symptoms for a few hours the day after receiving their first treatment with Aredia or Zometa, but these symptoms rarely occur after the first administration.

Not only can we reduce the occurrence of bone-related problems with drugs like bisphosphonates, but we also know that simply taking vitamin D and calcium can help. The amount of vitamin D that most people receive daily, about 400-800 international units, is often inadequate for myeloma patients. Many patients are deficient. Thus, measurement of vitamin D levels in the blood should be done at diagnosis and every 6–12 months thereafter. If it is low, once-weekly higher doses of 50,000 international units are required for about two months, at which time a repeat blood test should be performed to make sure that an adequate level has been reached. Although myeloma patients may develop high calcium levels in the blood when the bone loss is severe, most patients need calcium supplements in the amount of one gram daily. Monitoring of blood calcium levels is important since if the levels do become high, both vitamin D, which increases calcium levels, and calcium supplements should be discontinued.

In addition to medical management with treatment using drugs and vitamins, we also may have you seen by an orthopedic or back surgeon. They can help assess your bone disease. Does it need surgical intervention and the help of a physical therapist or rehab medicine doctor? Remember the oncologists and hematologists are trained in bone marrow-related diseases, but not in bone-related disorders—that often requires the expertise of an orthopedic or back surgeon. We also believe that staying active is very important. Weight-bearing exercise keeps your bones in good shape, reducing the chance of you experiencing bone-related problems and helping you maintain a healthy and happy lifestyle. Don't just lie around—that's how more bone loss occurs, resulting in both fractures and increased blood calcium levels, which can be a serious problem.

Thus, keeping your bones healthy and happy over the long run requires an integrative approach, not only involving treatment with drugs like bisphosphonates, supplements with adequate vitamin D, or minerals like calcium, but also often the involvement of an orthopedic or back surgeon, physical therapists, and rehabilitation medicine doctors. Occasionally, patients may need radiation therapy to relieve bone pain or treat fractures, but this is being used less often today with the effective use of bisphosphonates and other interventions that are now available through your oncologist, including effective treatment of the myeloma to eliminate the cause of bone loss, as well as the help of orthopedic and back surgical colleagues. Radiation therapy may have serious side effects, including further compromising the patient's bone marrow function, which may compromise administration of treatment for the myeloma.

Anemia

It's likely that sometime during the course of your myeloma that you are going to become anemic. So, what is anemia? It means your red blood cell count is low. So, what does that do to you if your red cell count is low? Well, red cells carry oxygen, so if you don't have enough oxygen, as you know, you're going to feel weak and tired. So, we're going to do everything we can to prevent that. But, it turns out there may be a lot of reasons why that may occur in a myeloma patient. It could be the myeloma itself is making it so you can't grow red cells in your bone marrow. After all, the red cells are made there, and the myeloma cells are lurking there. They may shut off your ability to make red cells if they crowd out the bone marrow. It could be treatment, chemotherapy, or radiation shuts off your red cell production. It also may be that your kidneys are not functioning properly from your myeloma or other causes. Since the growth protein that we call erythropoietin, or EPO, for red cell production is produced in the kidney, compromised kidney function can also compromise production of this red cell growth factor. Without this factor, you're going to become anemic.

So, how do we monitor you for anemia? We simply measure the number of red cells in your blood. These blood tests include your hemoglobin, your hematocrit, or your RBC count. If the count is low enough, we're going to want to either transfuse you, or we're going to give you some supplements to help you prevent anemia. The best one we have right now is called EPO. This is in two forms today, either Aranesp or Procrit. And these can boost your hemoglobin level.

But we've also learned over the last several years that many patients with myeloma are iron- or vitamin B12-deficient. Measurement of vitamin B12 and iron levels should be done if you are, in fact, anemic. Bone marrow exams will also assess iron stores. If iron or vitamin B12 deficiency is identified, simply giving Procrit or Aranesp will not improve the anemia. You will need iron as well, specifically intravenously administered iron. Vitamin B12 can also be given if you are deficient. Even if you are not found to be low on these measurements at their first assessment, this may occur over time, so repeat levels should be measured periodically, especially if your anemia persists. If the use of EPO, iron, and B12 does not work, you may require transfusions of red cells. This may eventually lead you to become iron overloaded. This can result in serious problems in your heart, liver, or other major organs. We have drugs to help with that, as well, especially one called Exjade.

Proper monitoring of your hemoglobin is a key to the long-term successful management of your multiple myeloma. Recently, there's been concern that the use of EPO for patients with myeloma and other cancers perhaps is actually speeding up the cancer's growth and shortening the survival of cancer patients. There are studies evaluating this; some have shown that's the case whereas others have not confirmed this.

You don't want to go overboard with the use of drugs like Procrit or Aranesp. Your doctor will work with you to make sure you're only receiving it when you absolutely need to. We want to make sure that you have proper levels of circulating red cells so you have good energy but we don't want to overdo it. So, make sure your doctors are measuring the hemoglobin level on a regular basis, and treating you with either drugs like Procrit or Aranesp, or if need be, transfusions. Maintaining your red cell count will help prevent you from being tired or unable to perform your work, and help you engage in the activities that you enjoy.

Kidney Disease

Another frequent problem with your myeloma involves its negative impact on your kidneys. This may be from the myeloma cells attacking the kidney, which is actually uncommon, or more likely from three other causes: the monoclonal antibody produced by the cancer cells being toxic to the kidney, high calcium levels in the blood, which can impact the kidney, or breakdown products of the monoclonal protein called amyloid. All of these problems may lead to kidney disease, but also there may be drugs you are receiving for the myeloma, drugs like the bisphosphonates, antibiotics, or other treatments, that impact the kidneys. Reducing the risk involves effective treatment of the myeloma while making sure you're receiving the proper doses of drugs. You may have to reduce the dose of many drugs if your kidney function is not normal. You also have to make sure the drugs you're receiving are not ones that put you at additional risk of developing kidney problems. Frequently myeloma patients may have other diseases that cause kidney problems like diabetes or hypertension, so it's important to make sure those are in control so they're not negatively impacting your kidneys even more than simply from the myeloma itself. Drugs you may be receiving for other diseases may also place added pressure on your kidneys and reduce their function.

In order to reduce the impact of kidney disease, it's important that you see a kidney specialist if you have abnormal kidney function. They help a lot with management of your fluids, phosphate levels, and other minerals that may be impacted by kidney function. We don't want you to end up on dialysis. Another important point is that you need to keep yourself well hydrated. Lots of fluid is a key, and minimizing dehydration will reduce your risk of ever having a kidney problem. Overall, kidney disease occurs commonly at some point during the course of a myeloma patient's disease. The good news is that today with all of the highly effective therapies, chances are good that your kidney function will improve, and as it does in many cases, get back to normal.

Nerve Problems

Nervous system problems commonly occur in myeloma patients. The drugs we use may affect the central nervous system; drugs like thalidomide may make you sleepy. More frequently these problems involve your peripheral nervous system, which is made up of the nerves that innervate your hands, feet, arms, and legs. Often patients develop peripheral neuropathies: numbness, tingling, and, less often, pain in their hands and feet. This may be from the monoclonal antibodies themselves that are made by the malignant plasma cells; they can coat the nerves and make them not function properly. But more frequently today the medications we use to treat the myeloma are the culprits, drugs like Velcade and thalidomide. The treatment of peripheral neuropathy may involve drugs such as Neurontin or the more recently developed drug Lyrica. Other drugs used include Cymbalta and doxepin. In addition, over-the-counter medications may help. We often use alpha-lipoic acid. This helps to reduce the occurrence and severity of peripheral neuropathy.

Now, in addition to the drug-induced neuropathy, we also know that certain anti-myeloma drugs can cause viral infections that are associated with nerve problems, such as shingles, caused by the herpes zoster virus. This is the reactivation of the chicken pox virus and presents often as a painful skin rash on one side of the body. For patients who are receiving drugs like arsenic or the proteasome inhibitors Velcade or Kyprolis, we may prescribe acyclovir or other drugs that are anti-herpetic, as long as they remain on these anti-myeloma drugs.

It's very important to let your doctor know if you're experiencing any problems with your nerves, especially if you're on drugs that may be causing it. Your doctor may want to intervene with drugs and may want to reduce the dosage of the drugs you are receiving or stop them altogether. Communication is the key that will allow you to reap the long-term benefits from the drugs you're receiving for myeloma while minimizing their side effects, which may not be reversible if the drug isn't discontinued or reduced in dosage soon enough.

FAQ 19: What Are Other Conditions That Are Similar to Multiple Myeloma?

Waldenstrom's Macroglobulinemia

This is an uncommon form of lymphoma that involves cancer cells that are quite similar to the type found in multiple myeloma. Patients are often discovered to have the disease when they are found to have high protein levels from the excessive amount of IgM antibody on routine blood tests. These high levels of IgM can occasionally cause a condition called hyperviscosity in which the blood is too thick from the excessive amount of antibody. This can lead to damage of many organs, including the kidney, brain, and heart. Occasionally, patients may have enlarged lymph nodes or spleen. Recently, a specific mutation in a gene called MYD88 has been identified in most patients with macroglobulinemia. Importantly, many patients never require treatment for this condition. When therapy is required, the treatments that are used are quite similar to those used for both myeloma and lymphoma, including Rituxan, also known as rituximab, an antibody treatment commonly used to treat lymphoma. Recently, two other drugs, Ibruvica, also known as ibrutinib, and Zydelig, also known as idelalisib, that have shown high levels of activity in lymphoma and a common form of leukemia, chronic lymphocytic leukemia, have been shown to also be very effective for treating patients with Waldenstrom's macroglobulinemia. Ibruvica inhibits a protein called Bruton tyrosine kinase, and Zydelig blocks PI3kinase activity. Because macroglobulinemia patients respond to drugs used to treat both lymphoma and multiple myeloma, these patients have more treatment options available than patients with either of these other similar types of cancer. Sometimes the condition becomes a more aggressive form of lymphoma that can be difficult to control. In general, most patients with Waldenstrom's macroglobulinemia are able to live long and productive lives often not requiring therapy or, if so, for only short periods of time.

Light Chain Amyloidosis

Light chain amyloidosis is a relatively uncommon disorder in which patients have depositing in organs of a part of a protein that turns out to be a breakdown product of the same antibody protein that is the marker for myeloma. This is caused by the inability of the protein to be broken down in such a fashion that it can be removed from the body. The patients often present without symptoms or may present with symptoms related to the accumulation of the amyloid protein in different organs. Specifically, they may develop shortness of breath, tiredness, weight loss, bleeding problems, swelling, high levels of protein in their urine, low blood pressure, nerve problems, diarrhea, or constipation. On physical examination, they may have enlarged tongues from the deposition of the amyloid protein there. Many different organs may be involved in patients with amyloidosis, although the kidneys, nervous system, and heart are the most common sites impacted. The goal of treatment is to remove the offending protein by getting rid of the plasma cells that are producing it, the monoclonal antibody and its amyloid-causing breakdown product, in the bone marrow. As a result, these patients are treated quite similarly to myeloma. It is important to recognize, though, that patients may have specific amyloid-related heart problems that require additional close follow-up. Unfortunately, patients with heart involvement do quite poorly in general.

Patients with kidney involvement, which also occurs frequently in amyloidosis, generally do well, although some may develop dialysis-dependent kidney failure. Patients with nerve disease from the depositing of the protein in the nerves may have numbness and tingling and may benefit from not only treating and getting rid of the protein by eliminating the plasma cells but from other drugs that may help as well (see section above on Nerve Problems). Some patients are treated with either autologous transplant or, rarely, allogeneic transplant. Even heart or kidney transplants are performed sometimes for patients with more severe disease.

The greatly increasing number of new therapies available for myeloma patients have also shown effectiveness in amyloid patients, and greatly improved their outcomes. Recently, attempts have been made to remove the amyloid protein from the affected organs, and early results from clinical trials are promising. Because of this and advances in the treatment of multiple myeloma, it is expected that patients with amyloidosis will be able to look forward to marked improvement in their lives.

Monoclonal Gammopathy of Undetermined Significance (MGUS)

Monoclonal gammopathy of undetermined significance, otherwise known as MGUS, is a disorder of the same type of white cell that is abnormal in myeloma, the plasma cell. However, these patients have a lower number of bone marrow plasma cells, less than 10%, and they also have smaller protein peaks of the monoclonal type, less than 3g/dl, and they do not have the end organ damage characteristic of myeloma, or the bone disease, kidney problems, high calcium, or anemia.

The frequency of MGUS is fairly high. Studies done in Olmsted County, where the Mayo Clinic is located, have shown that 3% of people over 50, 5% of people over 70, and 9% of people over 85 have this disorder. It is also more common in African-Americans than Caucasians. These patients do not require treatment, except if they have bone disease as evidenced by bone loss on bone density studies. This occurs frequently in this population and those patients should be treated with anti-bone loss therapy with drugs such as Zometa or Aredia every six months.

It is important to realize that patients with MGUS have a higher risk of developing multiple myeloma, with the risk being about 1% per year in general. Patients with higher levels of the monoclonal protein as well as patients who have an abnormal serum free light chain level in the blood have a greater chance of developing myeloma or related diseases such as lymphoma. It has also been shown that patients who have a non-IgG type that is IgM, IgA, or light chain type, are at high risk as well. It is also important to recognize that if patients have higher levels of normal antibodies (for example if they have an IgG monoclonal protein, and their IgM and IgA levels are in the normal range), they would be at lower risk.

It is also important to recognize that MGUS patients are at higher risk not only for bone disease but peripheral neuropathy, as well as having blood clots and infections. These patients may also have a slightly higher risk of cancer in general.

The management of patients with MGUS generally just involves following them with periodic labs every 6 to 12 months, although if they have bone loss they should be treated for that condition with anti-bone loss drugs such as Zometa or Aredia approximately every 6 months.

Summary

Treatment of myeloma and related conditions such as primary amyloidosis and Waldenstrom's macroglobulinemia is often a balancing act between the benefits of treatment versus its untoward side effects. It is important for drugs to be used at effective doses that are well tolerated, especially when used in combination with one another. It is important to keep in mind that many of the newer agents can be used effectively at lower doses and at the same time also allow the use of older agents such as chemotherapy or steroids to be used at lower doses.

Moreover, supportive care for bone disease, anemia, and kidney problems with drugs, supplements, physical therapy, and surgery can often greatly improve the quality of life of our patients. As patients are now living longer lives with these disorders, we must keep in mind that their quality of life now takes on even more importance. Side effects that we did not observe with shorter lifespans in the past are now being identified and potentially become part of our patient's burden as they live longer and longer. Our job is making sure we keep these side effects to a minimum without compromising our patients' overall lifespan with these diseases.

You Have…

MULTIPLE MYELOMA!

WALDENSTROM'S MACROGLOBULINEMIA!

AMYLOIDOSIS!

MGUS!

(Monoclonal Gammopathy of Undetermined Significance)

By Anne Meyer, MD -- (PM&R)

Diplomat, American Academy

of Physical Medicine & Rehabilitation

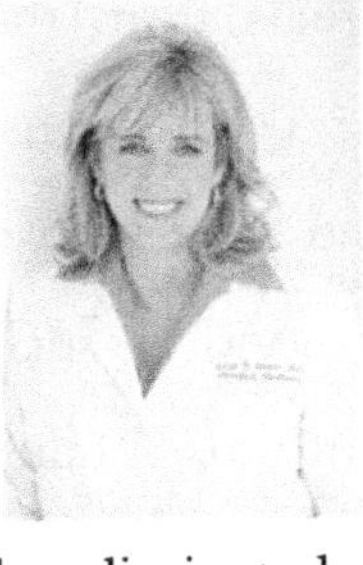

As a medical doctor specializing in Physical Medicine and Rehabilitation (PM&R), most of the people I meet in my office are referred for treatment of some type of musculoskeletal pain. As you can imagine, pain isn't much fun. But it can be eliminated or at least well controlled so you can be active. Pain gets in the way of living. Most of us don't have time for it. In some cases, multiple myeloma presents with a compression fracture of the spine. OUCH! This is often successfully treated with a procedure called a "kyphoplasty," performed by a spine surgeon. But remember, besides the challenges that myeloma or the related bone disorders present, there are still the aches and pains that come along with just living an active life.

This is where my specialty, PM&R, is important to the team. I know that what you are dealing with makes that old achy shoulder injury from college or stiff low back from "whatever" seem inconsequential. But those prior issues still affect the way that you feel each day. One thing I can say for sure is that the patients who come to me from Dr. James Berenson for help with pain management or rehabilitation are very special indeed. I recognize a strength and confidence that comes from within you, as well as from knowing you are part of Dr. Berenson's team of healthcare professionals. These qualities support you in your commitment to an individual plan that will optimize your comfort and energy.

I believe it is important to identify each patient's goals from the beginning. Understanding your lifestyle, social connections, responsibilities, problems, and habits are all critical parts of a successful game plan. We are all multi-faceted beings, and as such there are many ways to approach the journey to health. Taking inventory of your life may seem daunting but breaking it down into slices is easy.

- From the thoughts we entertain to the company we keep, our minds can assist or resist our recovery. Surround yourself with affirmative words and people.
- Honoring your body by consuming whole live foods that resemble a plant, rather than have been manufactured in a plant, is a great step to take. Knowing what foods fuel you and what foods to eliminate, because they are inflammatory, is vital. Foods should recharge us.
- Your body needs restorative sleep. It always did, but now it is most essential. Healing and repair take place during sleep. Knowing proper sleep hygiene tips can help you get eight hours per night of uninterrupted sleep. Tips such as unplugging yourself from all electronic gadgets (television, computer) for at least one hour before bedtime. Use black-out curtains or a sleep mask to prevent your brain from perceiving light before you wake up. Melatonin and growth hormone are both produced during sleep—when your brain is not exposed to light. Try closing your eyes right now. Unless you are in a pitch black room, you are aware of light through your eyelids. Ask yourself if you can see the furniture in your room when you wake up in the morning. If the answer if "yes," then your brain did not have true black-out for the entire time that you were sleeping. This will impact your production of melatonin (the sleep/wake cycle hormone), as well as the amount of growth hormone which is important for muscle strength. Try a warm Epsom salt

bath and use therapeutic grade essential oils such as lavender or valerian on your feet before slipping between the percales.

- Exercise that you enjoy and can perform not only ramps up your natural endorphins (the happy molecules) but will help boost your strength and immune system too. You can learn what activities work best for you and do them at your pace.
- Hydration with pure water is so important! Your body will thank you. If you just thought to yourself "I'm probably not drinking enough," you are probably correct. Hydration with WATER helps to decrease muscle soreness, stiffness, headaches, and irritability. You cannot have a deficiency of diet soda.
- For treatment of musculoskeletal pain, I use techniques such as acupuncture, homeopathy, tailored exercises, kinesiotaping, and trigger point injections using safe solutions that target inflammation without the side effects of steroids. If needed, steroids can be used, but I find that utilizing the above mentioned methods may be just the ticket. Environmental assessments of movement incorporating good biomechanics and ergonomics can often reveal sources (usually habits) that aggravate pain. Modifying these may be a simple solution to feeling better.

Along with optimal nutrition, hydration, sleep, and exercise for repair and strength, I believe we all should have our nutrient levels evaluated. There are specialty labs that can provide us with this data.

Measuring our current nutrient levels can help to provide us with a roadmap to determine which supplements need to be replenished.

Nature has provided us with many answers. It is my belief that we need to listen. With all the physical challenges you are going through with treatment for multiple myeloma or its related disorders, taking time out each day to appreciate small things can have a huge positive impact on how you feel. Remember, we can choose how we react to anything. This is very empowering. And one more thing…you are more than this diagnosis.

You Have…

MULTIPLE MYELOMA!

WALDENSTROM'S MACROGLOBULINEMIA!

AMYLOIDOSIS!

MGUS!

(Monoclonal Gammopathy of Undetermined Significance)

By Benjamin M. Eades, -- Pharm Tech

Director of Pharmacy

James R. Berenson MD, Inc.

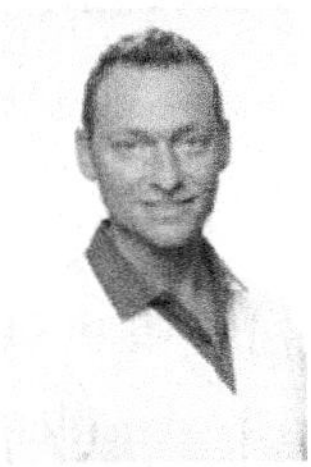

I have managed the clinic pharmacy at Dr. Berenson's practice for nine years. My daily duties include preparing chemotherapy medication orders, calculating drug dosages, drug inventory, investigational and clinical trial drug accountability, mixing chemotherapy treatments, checking patient medication lists for contra-indications, and counseling patients on their current regimens.

Working for a world-renowned specialist in myeloma has been an amazing experience thus far. I have had the opportunity to meet hundreds of patients from around the world and prepare recommended drug treatment regimens tailored to suit each patient's specific needs based on their renal function, cardiac history, nerve problems, etc. I will then sit down and thoroughly explain each medication and its possible side effects, list medications and supplements to prevent or help with these side effects, and ensure that each patient has an understanding of the recommended regimen. A copy of the recommendation will also be sent to the patient's primary oncologist.

Most of Dr. Berenson's treatment regimens are very well tolerated with minimal side effects due to their longer cycles and lower doses than recommended in the information provided by the drug manufacturers. One class of drugs to treat myeloma is the proteasome inhibitors. Two drugs in this class approved to treat multiple myeloma include bortezomib and carfilzomib. One of the major side effects of this class of drug is peripheral neuropathy, a burning or tingling sensation usually felt in the hands or feet. Dr. Berenson has implemented the use of alpha-lipoic acid, an over-the-counter antioxidant, to prevent and treat existing peripheral neuropathy in patients being treated with this class of drug. Another side effect of proteasome inhibitors can be a shingles outbreak. To prevent this, an oral antiviral drug such as acyclovir or valacyclovir is prescribed to be taken daily while on the regimen containing the proteasome inhibitor and for up to six to eight weeks after stopping the regimen. We observe nausea and vomiting infrequently with the doses of drugs used in our clinic, but antiemetic drugs are available if needed to control these symptoms. Some patients receive an injection of palonosetron to control the nausea for up to seven days, or some prefer taking oral drugs such as ondansetron, granisetron, or prochlorperazine. Blood clots can occur among patients who are taking the class of drug known as immunomodulatory agents. Drugs in this class include lenalidomide, thalidomide, and pomalidomide. A baby aspirin taken orally daily is recommended by Dr. Berenson to keep the blood thin enough to prevent clotting unless the patient has additional risk factors for developing blood clots.

One other class of drugs taken by myeloma patients is bisphosphonates. Zoledronic acid and pamidronate are two examples of this drug class used in our clinic. Bones are constantly building new cells (osteoblasts) and breaking down old cells (osteoclasts). Bisphosphonates disrupt this homeostasis and inhibit the breakdown of healthy bone, thereby slowing down bone loss, which occurs at an accelerated rate in myeloma patients. Some patients experience flu-like symptoms with the first few infusions of these drugs. The side effects are usually managed by taking acetaminophen before the infusion. There is also a possibility of osteonecrosis of the jaw (ONJ) with bisphosphonates. It is very important to have regular dental examinations and hold bisphosphonate treatments before and after major dental work such as extractions. Rarely, kidney problems can develop from these drugs, but checking the patient's kidney function prior to each infusion and maintaining hydration can help reduce the occurrence of this complication.

With certain chemotherapeutic agents, some side effects can't be avoided, such as thrombocytopenia (low platelet counts), neutropenia (low white blood cell counts), or anemia (low red blood cell counts). Fortunately, there is a rest period with each regimen of at least one week that allows the body to build these levels back up before starting the next round. Sometimes, if the numbers drop too low, transfusions are needed, but most of the time a simple injection such as epoetin alfa or filgrastim can give the cells a needed boost.

Dr. Berenson is at the forefront of research and development of new myeloma treatment regimens. I feel very fortunate to be a part of his research team, who has had numerous articles published in medical magazines and journals and combinations of drugs approved for myeloma therapy. I have been involved in more than 30 studies and trials since I joined the team. We currently have 10 active studies and many more on the way. I look forward to continuing to educate patients on their regimens and being on this amazing team of medical professionals that is searching for a cure.

You Have…

MULTIPLE MYELOMA!

WALDENSTROM'S MACROGLOBULINEMIA!

AMYLOIDOSIS!

MGUS!

(Monoclonal Gammopathy of Undetermined Significance)

By Edward J. Share, MD -- Gastroenterologist

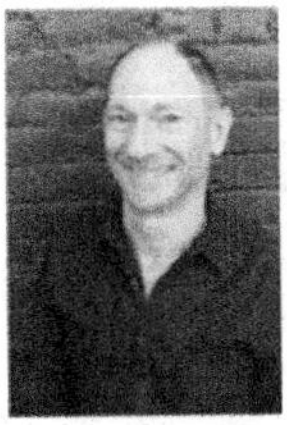

When I'm asked to see a patient with multiple myeloma or other plasma cell disorders, it is usually because they have constipation, abdominal pain, or anemia with a drop in blood count.

Constipation can be defined as infrequent or hard stools. It is worthy of attention if the sluggish bowel habit is causing symptoms, including abdominal discomfort, bloating, or fullness in the abdomen. Rectal bleeding may also be associated with constipation when hard stools irritate the hemorrhoidal veins at the bottom of the rectum. In fact, constipation is one of the most common causes of abdominal pain that we gastroenterologists see.

A number of medications used to treat myeloma often cause constipation by interfering with the normal colon motility function. Revlimid and Velcade are medications that often do this. This side effect needs to be ameliorated so that patients may be continued on these highly effective myeloma drugs.

The colon's function is to receive liquid waste from the small intestine and move it along by peristaltic contractions (like a snake that swallows a frog) while it reabsorbs water and electrolytes. Harder stools and narrower stools are more difficult to push along than more bulky, softer stools. The first line of therapy for constipation includes stool-bulking agents and stool-softening agents. Stool-bulking agents include high fiber morning cereals such as Fiber One (14gm) and All-Bran (10gm) as well as psyllium (Metamucil) and guar gum (Benefiber). A very effective stool softener is mineral oil and it can be found in a preparation called Kondremul that combines mineral oil with a natural bulking agent called Irish Moss, as well as a small amount of marshmallow for taste. This is taken at bedtime in a dose of 1–3 tablespoons. Other softeners and bulking agents are available, and there are prescription medications that soften stools by stimulating the secretion of water across the small intestine and colon lining cells into the lumen (inside) of the bowel, such as Amitiza and Linzess. Stimulant laxatives are quite effective in the short run but are best avoided when possible because they lead to resistance, with the need for ever-increasing doses until they eventually may not work at all. These include senna, cascara, cape aloe leaf, and laxative or herbal teas.

To achieve an effective regimen requires regular communication between the patient and physician and is required in order to continue effective myeloma therapy.

Anemia (low red blood cell count) due to bone marrow suppression of the formation of these red cells is a common side effect of the numerous chemotherapeutic agents needed to achieve remission in myeloma. This cause of anemia must be differentiated from the silent loss of these red cells from the gastrointestinal tract as a result of slow (occult) bleeding. Such blood loss if chronic over months can lead to loss of the iron in these cells and thus "iron deficiency anemia." Ulcers in the stomach or first part of the small intestine (duodenum) can be caused by medications such as Advil and aspirin, even in small doses if used on a daily basis. Slow blood loss from these ulcers or "erosions" in the upper GI tract is best evaluated by an "Upper Gastrointestinal Endoscopy" where one is sedated and has a thin "scope" passed through the mouth into the stomach. Colonoscopy is also advised to insure there is no bleeding source in the lower intestine (colon). If these are both negative, a "wireless capsule enteroscopy" may be performed. In this study, a small camera inside of a capsule the size of a vitamin is swallowed and passes through the small intestine. Over 8–12 hours, it records images that are transmitted to a device one wears that day. Bleeding and/or abnormalities in the 15–20 feet of small intestine can be seen and, if present, may be further evaluated with scopes that can visualize the small intestine. One can test the stools for blood with a chemical test to see if there is evidence of blood loss through the stool, but this may be intermittent and the above careful evaluation is commonly performed.

On occasion, an iron deficiency anemia is present but no abnormality is found. In this situation, the doctor may administer intravenous iron to replace the low iron stores, but be reassured that there is no significant problem that needs immediate treatment. Poor absorption of iron may be the source of that situation but is hard to prove! Abdominal pain can be caused by a very diverse list of problems and certainly needs to be expeditiously evaluated. The "history" given to a gastroenterologist is often the best clue to the source of the problem and is the first "test" that may be done. Often, constipation is the problem. But any of the organs in the abdomen or pelvis may be the culprit, and imaging of this area is extremely helpful. CT scanning ("computerized tomography") is a quick, non-invasive X-ray that is quite accurate in visualizing the "tubular GI tract" from stomach to rectum as well as the gallbladder, liver, pancreas, and what's in between, like the mesentery and lymph nodes. MRI (magnetic resonance imaging) uses a magnet rather than X-ray and may be helpful to home in on a specific organ, or can be used instead of CT imaging in certain situations. Of course, if an ulcer is suspected, the upper GI endoscopy is the procedure of choice. Barium X-rays such as Upper GI series and Barium Enema are mostly procedures of the past but on rare occasion may be useful.

These gastrointestinal problems can almost always be solved, allowing life-saving therapy to continue. The key is to remember you're in this for the long run and to not allow these bumps in the road to knock you off your game. There will be side effects that will be treated and unexpected roadblocks. But with courage, confidence you will prevail, and with a solid team behind you, you will succeed!

As one of my colleagues explained to me, "We all have something"... We do the best we can!

You Have…

MULTIPLE MYELOMA!

WALDENSTROM'S MACROGLOBULINEMIA!

AMYLOIDOSIS!

MGUS!

(Monoclonal Gammopathy of Undetermined Significance)

By Ian A. Novotny, PT, DPT -- Physical Therapist

Back2Health Physical Therapy

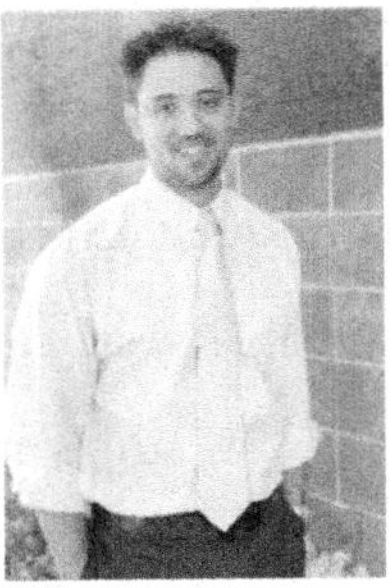

What is physical therapy and can it help me?

Thanks to the amazing work that Dr. Berenson is doing, people with multiple myeloma are not only living longer, but living more fruitful lives. The goal of physical therapy is to reduce the impact that the symptoms associated with multiple myeloma have on the way you feel and improve your productivity, activity levels, and participation in life. Physical therapists use exercise, special machines that increase circulation and reduce pain, and manual techniques to improve strength, flexibility, posture, coordination, endurance, and tolerance to activity. They can give you advice about how to be active, how to make the most of the energy you have, and how to protect yourself from injury. These specialists design patient- specific plans for exercise, treatment, and patient education to improve your quality of life.

Therapeutic Exercise

Exercising while supervised by a physical therapist ensures that you are performing safe, low-impact exercises with the correct alignment to promote health, wellness, and functional performance. The importance of safety when exercising is magnified by the decrease in bone density associated with multiple myeloma. Performing exercise correctly can be greatly beneficial in improving bone density, but doing resisted activity with improper technique can lead to injury, increased joint stress, fractures, and even bone degeneration. We will make sure you do the right exercises, in the right way. You can be active and energized with the confidence that you are doing the best things for your physical wellbeing. Physical Therapists understand the specific symptoms and risks associated with your condition and can guide you through a routine that helps to build strength, improve balance, and increase endurance.

Manual Treatment

Most of our patients with multiple myeloma complain of joint stiffness, muscle tension, and reduced tolerance to movement. While this is caused by the cells affected by the disease and the drugs used to treat it, you can still do something to reduce these symptoms. Physical therapists can perform and teach you how to perform gentle massage on stiff joints and tense muscles. Through stretching and joint mobilization, the tissue around your joints can move more easily. You can get the mobility in your body so you can climb stairs, hike, swim, get up from a low couch, play golf, even ski, and enjoy your family. Massage increases circulation, bringing nutrients and oxygen to the muscles, bones and joints. It also helps to wash out the chemicals and waste byproducts in your body that create pain. It warms and preconditions the tissue to stretch and glide during movement. It helps you produce the natural lubricants in the joints to ease movement.

Dr. Berenson described the cellular mechanics causing bone pain. When you have pain, the body tries to protect itself by contracting the muscles around the joints to reduce movement. This is called muscle guarding, and it is why you may feel knots in the muscles all over your body. This is a protective mechanism that is a reflex. The body thinks that if it limits movement, it can reduce potential damage that could cause more pain. The problem with this is that muscle spasm decreases blood flow to working muscles as well as restricting movement. This reduction in blood flow deprives the area of oxygen and nutrition, actually causing more pain because the tissue is actually starving! The result is what we call a pain-spasm cycle. The pain causes muscle spasm in order to guard the area; the spasm causes pain due to lack of circulation resulting in more pain; and the cycle repeats. Through manual techniques, we can release the knots in your muscles and reduce the spasm to break the pain-spasm cycle.

Patient Education

One of the most important things physical therapists can help you with is to understand how multiple myeloma affects your function. I find that most of my patients have fears about how to get through the day. How can you accomplish daily tasks when you are tired and in pain? Two principles of patient education that we use in the clinic to help people become more productive are joint protection and energy conservation.

Joint protection deals with habits and techniques you can use to reduce the stress to your joints. Decreasing joint stress will help to reduce the intensity of pain and the frequency of potential fractures. First, use larger joints. When you have the option, lift or carry with the large joints in the legs and shoulders rather than the small joints of the hands and spine. You've heard people say, "Lift with your legs." This means that you are using the big, strong muscles in the glutes, hamstrings, and quads to move and lift things. When you do this, you should keep your back straight. When you bend, you should feel the bend in the hips and knees. Remember to squat to pick up objects rather than bending at your spine. If your chest is up, then your spine is usually straight. When stirring the pot while cooking, move your whole arm instead of just the wrist. Use built- up grips on utensils and pens. When you spread the force out over a larger surface area, you feel less pain. If you open the door, use your legs to push your hip into it instead of the hands. When you pick up objects with the palm down, you have to use the fingers. Instead, pick up objects with your palm facing up. This ensures you are using the big, strong bicep muscles in your arms instead of the small muscles and joints of the hands.

Instead of carrying objects, use rolling carts to transport items. One of the smartest patients I've had used a rolling wooden cart in the kitchen to move pots and pans from the sink to the stove. The cart had wheels and a flat top, which doubled as a small island in her kitchen. If you have to carry a bag, place the handles over your forearm to carry small bags. Larger bags can go over the shoulder, saving the hands. Even better would be to use a backpack with two straps over the shoulders instead of just one. Again, spreading out the force reduces the stress you feel.

Joint protection is not restricted to the daytime. One of the most common questions patients have for me is "What is the best position to sleep in?" You basically have three positions to choose from: on your back, on your side, or on your stomach. Keep in mind that you are stuck in that position for hours at a time. There are two types of stress that build with time to consider, compression and sustained stretch. Bend your index finger back until you feel a stretch near the palm at the base of the finger. This may feel good at first, but keep holding the finger back. Continue reading while stretching your finger and we will come back to that in a second. The tissues in our bodies do not like to be compressed for prolonged periods. This restricts blood flow, crushes nerves, and limits expansion of the rib cage for breathing. Conversely, having tissue stretched for hours at a time is no picnic either. How is that finger of yours? Has it started to burn yet? We have only held the stretch for a minute, and maybe you have already given up. Now imagine stretching your finger for two, three, even eight hours! If your joints are not in a midline or neutral position, then you are stretching them for hours at a time. Of course, you wake with soreness and stiffness. So, sleep position can have an enormous impact on how we feel each day.

Sleeping flat on your back with one pillow is the ideal position from a joint and circulation standpoint. This places the joints in the most neutral position possible. The legs and arms are straight, the neck and back is in midline, and the pelvis is level. It allows the ribs to expand so you can breathe freely. The worst position is sleeping on your stomach. Your feet are pointed down and turned out, causing your legs to be twisted. The weight of your body is on the ribs, limiting chest expansion for breathing. Your arms are pushed back behind you, under the pillow, or over your head, causing pinching at the shoulders and that sustained stretch we just discussed. Then, unless you sleep with a snorkel, you head is turned to one side, causing compression on one side of the neck and sustained stretch to the other. Sleeping on your stomach is clearly in last place when choosing sleep position. In a distant second place, sleeping on your side presents some problems that can at least be reduced with pillows and positioning. If you are a side sleeper, you need to fill the space between your shoulder and your head. This usually requires two pillows or a pillow folded in half. If you fill this space, you can at least keep the neck in close to a midline position. Keep in mind that all of the weight of your body is still on one shoulder and one hip. By placing a pillow between your knees, you can keep the legs from crossing and twisting your spine. At least the ankles and feet are neutral in side lying.

Sleeping on your back is the easiest way to stay neutral, so if you are able to, you should try to change your sleep position. Sleep position can be learned, like anything else. To do this, start out in the desired position. If you wake, return to the desired position. Repeat to yourself before you fall asleep, "Wake up if I roll over, wake up if I roll over." If you get this in your subconscious, your body will wake when you move out of the desire position. If you sleep with someone, have them wake you when they see you in a poor position. With practice, your body will become more comfortable in the desired position, so don't give up. It literally will not change overnight!

Energy conservation does not mean you do nothing! By being smarter, you can be more active. Think of the total amount of energy you have each day as a dollar amount. You only have so much energy each day, so you can only spend so much. Patients with multiple myeloma are dealing with anemia, fatigue, kidney problems, nerve problems, bone pain, side effects of medication, stress, and shortness of breath. The frequent doctor visits alone to can be exhausting! So, you have to budget your energy. Planning your day can be the deciding factor in whether you get things done or have them pile up. You know what time of day you have the most energy. If you have more energy in the mornings and burnout by two p.m., then schedule your most important meetings in the mornings. Social activities can be at the top of the list, too! Tell your friends to meet for brunch instead of late-night dinners. Some of my patients take a few hours to get going each day, so later appointments suit them fine. You know your body, so plan accordingly.

Planning also deals with prioritizing. You may not get to every task each day. Try to tackle the most important duties first. If possible, combine your trips. This can be as simple as completing all the tasks you need to do upstairs before heading downstairs to the living room. If you reduce the trips up and down the stairs, you can use that energy on other tasks. When you leave the house, plan your route to make each stop flow into the next. Driving back and forth across town wastes time and energy.

Some tasks may be too big to complete in one day. So, try to break up the task into parts that you can do ahead of time. Suppose you have a big dinner party. Prepare the items you are cooking the night before. Cut up vegetables, make sauces, lay out the dishes, and decorate ahead of time. Use devices that do the work for you. Electric can openers, battery-powered wine corks, electric mixing bowls, and dishwashers were all invented to save you energy. Then you can plate the dishes and enjoy the party. Most importantly, you can enjoy your life! Not only will you get more done, but you will feel more alive.

Thermal Agents

Whether to use heat or ice is always a question that comes up when dealing with pain. Both heat and ice can help you in different ways. People have different reactions to heat and cold, so making one recommendation is difficult. I prefer to educate my patients on the potential benefits of each and suggest trying both. After a trial of each, use the one you seem to respond to. I usually recommend heating during the day and icing at night. Heat can be applied with moist heat packs, electrical heating pads, hot water bottles, and beanbags placed in the microwave. Taking hot baths or showers can help to reduce muscle spasm and tension. I recommend trying heat over muscular areas that are tight and tense and icing over joints that are swollen and inflamed. Warming tissue, as little as two degrees, increases local blood flow. We know circulation is important for bringing nutrients to working muscles, washing out chemicals that cause pain, and increasing tissue extensibility. As muscles and tendons warm up, they are easier to move. So, if you are moving and doing things, you should use heat. Some patients with multiple myeloma become heat sensitive due to the decrease in red blood cell count, decreased sensation associated with neuropathy, and the side effects from medication. Use towels between your skin and the hot pack to slow the warming effect and check your skin frequently until you have determined your response to heat. While increased circulation is important for nutrient delivery, it also can increase swelling due to the influx of blood. In those cases, icing may be indicated.

Icing is helpful for reducing local inflammation and swelling by vasoconstriction. When the area is cooled, the blood vessels contract, drawing the fluid in the area out of the periphery and effectively draining swollen, inflamed tissue. Many of our patients prefer icing because they often feel a burning sensation in their legs, hands, and feet. The cooling sensation can provide a respite from this sensation. One of the drawbacks of icing is that it may make you feel stiff. The most effective time to ice is right before bed. This is when your body may be the most swollen from the day's activity and the resulting stiffness will be less impactful since you won't be moving around.

Electrical stimulation

One of the machines we use in physical therapy to reduce pain is called *electrical stimulation.* Electrical stimulation uses sticky pads placed on the skin to run a current through the tissue to modulate pain, reduce muscle spasm, and help with healing. We have two pathways of nerves to the brain that deal with sensation. One is for light touch, and one is for pain. There is an interneuron in the brain that acts as a gate when the signals travel to the brain. Only one signal gets to go through the interneuron. The signal that arrives at the interneuron first goes on to the brain. Passage of the first signal closes the gate, reducing the perception of the second signal to reach the interneuron. Fortunately for us, the light touch pathway is faster to the brain than the pain pathway. So, when we stimulate the light touch pathway with electrical stimulation, more touch sensation is sent to the brain than pain. This is like when your mom would rub your knee when you fell off your bike as a kid. She is stimulating light touch pathway, so you feel less pain.

When you put your socks on in the morning, you feel them. After a little while, your brain says, okay that signal is not changing. So, it turns it off since no new information is coming in. This is called accommodation. When you place a constant stimulus into the body as with electrical stimulation, your nerves can effectively shut off the perception of signal in the area you have pain.

When I turn the machine on, you will first feel a tingling sensation called sensory level stimulation. As intensity increases, you may feel a twitching of the muscle called motor level stimulation. Muscle contraction occurs in the muscle cell based on a change in polarity, which is the same thing as an electrical current. Motor level stimulation can give you longer lasting pain relief by fatiguing out the muscle to reduce muscle spasm and increasing circulation through the pumping action of the muscle. We don't need to get to motor level stimulation, but it is not a bad thing if it is still comfortable.

There are portable electrical stimulation units called TENS (transcutaneous electrical nerve stimulation) units. These units can be purchased for home use, so you can have the benefits of pain management when you need it.

What symptoms can physical therapy help me with the most?

Bone Density

The primary musculoskeletal complication for people with multiple myeloma is loss of bone density. Bone density is dependent on two types of bone cells that constantly work in opposition. Osteoclasts remove and break down bone, whereas osteoblasts lay down new bone cells. Constant or repetitive stress stimulates osteoblast activity to increase the production of bone cells. More bone cells increases bone strength, thickness, and density. This stress is most effective in the form of weight bearing exercise, but can also be from muscles pulling on bones. Weight-bearing exercises include standing exercises as well as weight bearing on the arms, like a push-up or plank position.

The simplest weight-bearing exercise we use with our patients is called a "sit to stand" (*Figure 1*). This exercise can be performed anywhere with just a chair. Start by sitting on a stable chair. To perform correctly, place the feet shoulder width apart with the toes pointed straight forward. You can hold a weight in front of you to make the exercise more challenging. Keep your back straight, lean forward until you feel your bottom start to lift off the seat. Push your feet into the ground and come to a standing position. Watch your knees to make sure they stay directly on top of the feet without moving in front of the toes. Pull the weight to your chest as you stand. Slowly lower yourself to a sitting position while keeping your chest up. This exercise incorporates weight-bearing, a functional activity, like getting up from a chair, and alignment of the ankles, knees, and hips. The "sit to stand" is a safer form of a squat because you are less likely to move the knees into a damaging position and are able to keep the back straighter. Bone density has been shown to improve with as little as 12 to 20 minutes of exercise three times per week. Walking, stair climbing, weight lifting in standing, and sit to stands are just some weight-bearing exercises you can perform, but physical therapists can design a specific program for you to ensure your safety and maximize your bone density.

Figure 1.

SIT TO STAND

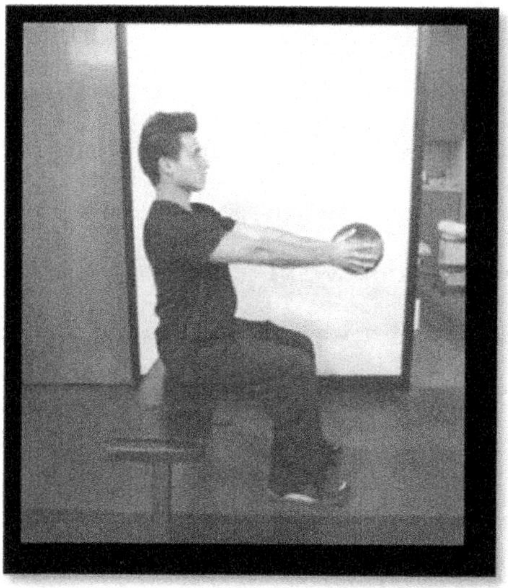

1. Begin in a seated position. Place the feet a shoulder width apart with the toes pointed forward. Keep the knees directly over the toes. Hold a ball or weight out in front of you.

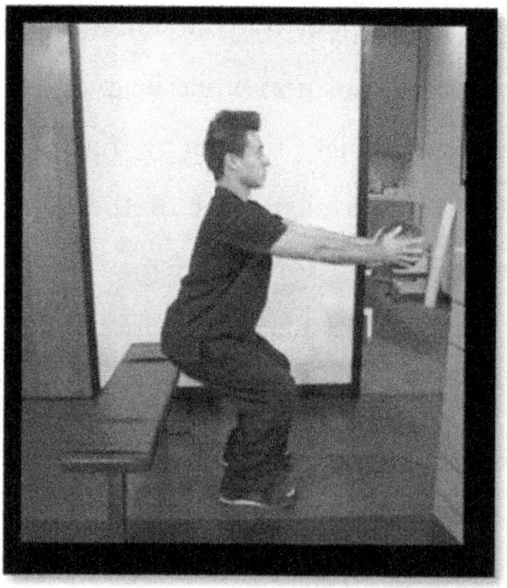

2. Lean your trunk forward, bending at the hips. Using your legs for power, press into the ground as you stand. Keep your chest up to maintain a neutral spine. Keep the knees in line, but behind the toes.

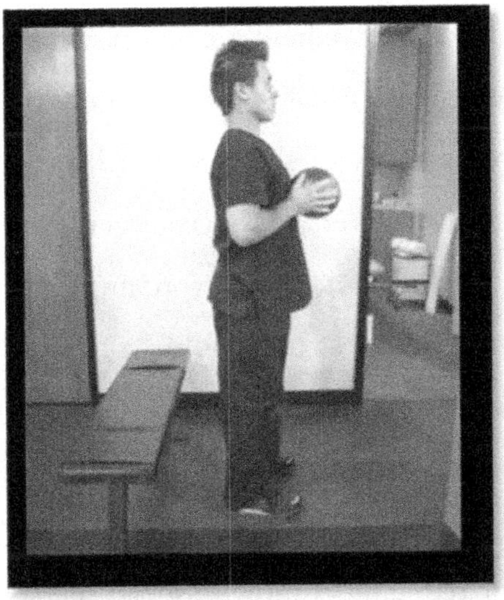

3. Bring the ball or weight into your chest as you stand.

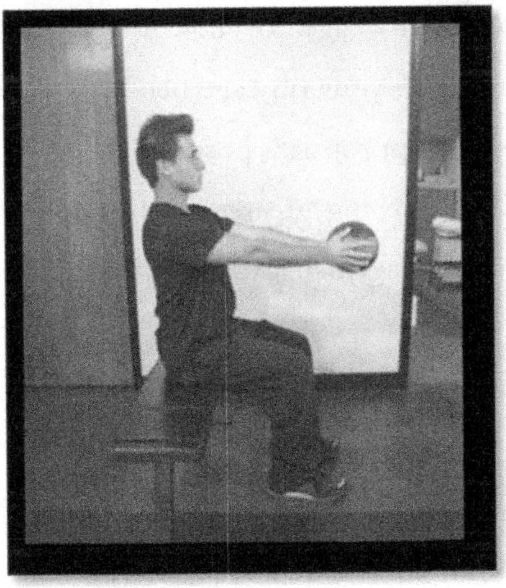

4. Slowly lower yourself to the chair, keeping the knees in line with the toes. Finish in a seated position with the ball out.

Posture

Spinal fractures are common among patients with multiple myeloma due to the lack of bone density. These fractures cause the bony blocks of the spine, called vertebral bodies, to collapse. This creates a painful, hunched posture as well as loss of height. This is often treated with a surgery called kyphoplasty, where a balloon is inserted into the vertebral body. The balloon re-inflates the segments of the spine, and cement is injected to restore the shape of the bones and stabilize the fracture. Regardless of whether you have surgery or treat these fractures conservatively, it is essential that you improve the strength and endurance of the muscles that hold you upright. Postural muscles have to work all day long to hold you upright against gravity. Gravity does not give up, so neither should you!

Upright posture is important for reducing compression on the spinal bones as well as opening up the rib cage to allow for improved breathing. As you breathe in and out, your rib cage needs to expand and contract. When you assume an appropriate posture, you increase the ability for the ribs to move, allowing greater expansion of the lungs. Improved breathing increases oxygen exchange, which helps you with our next symptom.

Fatigue

Anemia is a condition where you are lacking sufficient red blood cells to provide oxygen to the cells, organs, muscles, and tissues of the body. This insufficiency of red blood cells leads to significant fatigue because the muscles do not have the fuel to work. Through postural training, you can increase your body's ability to take in and transport oxygen to working muscles. Your body actually becomes more efficient at storing, transporting, and utilizing oxygen with regular exercise. I know you are not going to want to exercise. It is difficult to move and work against resistance when you are already exhausted. Our patients struggle the most with the initial session, but you will feel more energy if you keep trying. My best advice is to do what you can. You need to focus on what you can do, not what you can't do. A little is better than nothing, and the next time will be easier. Fatigue is a significant hurdle, but if you take steps, you will improve.

Weakness

One of the problems with fatigue is that it prevents you from doing things. We lose significant strength and even muscle mass in as little as two weeks of inactivity. Resisted exercise obviously restores and increases strength. Strength in the muscles is especially important for you because the muscles absorb the shock and stress of daily activities and walking. Strong muscles act as shock absorbers for the bones and joints. If you have decreased bone strength, strong muscles can prevent fractures. You need strength to maintain proper posture. You know you need weight-bearing exercise to improve bone density, so let's do it right. Shoulders back, chest up, knees in line with the toes, feet forward! Physical therapists will show you how to strengthen safely and with the proper alignment.

Neuropathy

Peripheral neuropathy is a common symptom in patients with multiple myeloma. Neuropathy is when the signal going to the muscles in the arms and legs is altered, causing pain, difficulty walking, decreased coordination, and weakness. The signal returning from the arms and legs is also diminished, resulting in numbness or a sensation of pins and needles. The neuropathy can be severe and sometimes debilitating. In multiple myeloma, peripheral neuropathy may be attributed to abnormal cell growth, mechanical compression of the nerves, or an autoimmune mechanism where the body is essentially attacking itself. There are many causes of neuropathy to occur in patients with multiple myeloma, but this may also be a side effect of the medications used to treat the myeloma. Examples of drugs causing treatment-related neuropathy include vincristine, platinum-containing agents (which are mostly of historic interest), thalidomide, and its newer derivatives lenalidomide and pomalidomide, and the proteasome inhibitor bortezomib as mentioned earlier by Dr. Berenson. With the advent of new drugs, the neurotoxicity caused by the medications prescribed has become a common cause of peripheral neuropathy. In evaluating the neuropathy, your physician typically performs electromyography and nerve conduction studies that measure the electrical integrity of the nerves to determine if the cause is chemical or mechanical, the location where the signal is disrupted, and the severity of the disruption.

If the neuropathy is caused by mechanical compression, physical therapists can show you how to take the physical pressure off the nerves. Imagine a garden hose with running water. When you step on the hose, it limits the flow of water. The same is true for nerve signals that run down to the hands and feet. Signals also run up from the periphery giving feedback like temperature, sensation, and where your limbs are positioned in space. Poor posture causes the bones to compress the space where nerves run, particularly by the spine. By improving posture, you can move the bones that may be pressing on the nerve, essentially taking your foot off the hose. Tight muscles can compress the nerve as well, so stretching helps to reduce the compression of nerves as they run through the limbs and improve the flow of signal down the nerves to the hands and feet. Additionally, physical therapists can show you exercises called nerve glides (Figure 2 and Figure 3). By moving your arms and legs in specific patterns, you can floss the nerve back and forth through the body. This frees up the nerve as it runs from the spine to the hands and feet. It also improves circulation to the nerve itself, improving the health of the nerve.

Figure 2.

UPPER EXTREMITY NERVE GLIDES

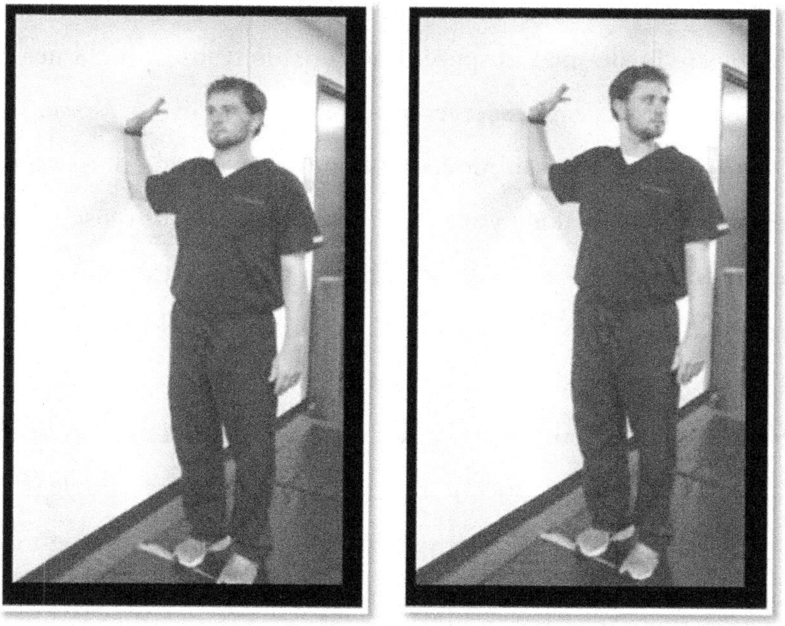

1. Place your forearm on the wall. Extend the wrist so your fingers are pointed at your head. Turn the head to the opposite side, looking away from the wall for 10 repetitions. Repeat on the opposite side.

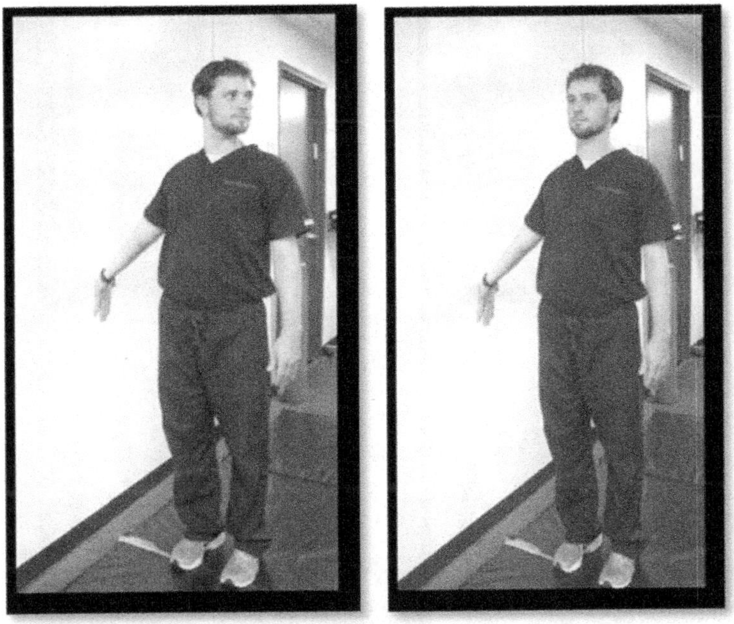

2. Place one hand on the wall with the fingers pointed down. Keeping the elbow straight, slide the hand up on the wall until you feel a stretch or pulling sensation. Turn the head to the opposite side, looking away from the wall for 10 repetitions. Repeat on the opposite side.

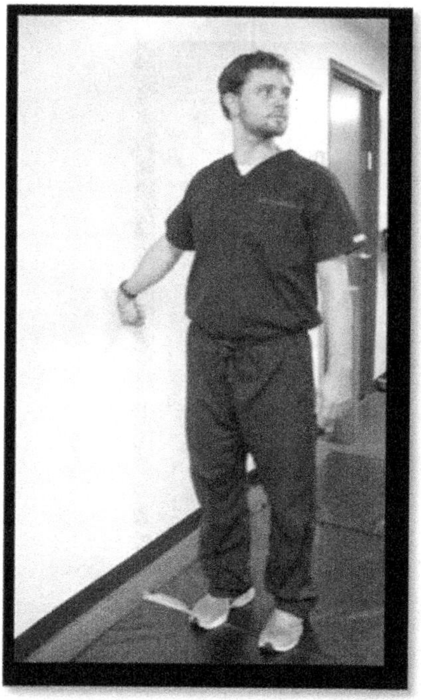

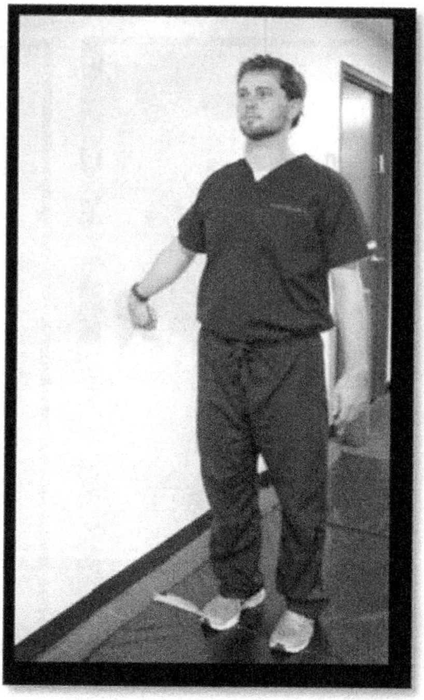

3. Make a fist with the thumb placed inside the hand. Place the knuckles of one hand on the wall. Rotate the hand forward like you are turning a door knob. To increase intensity, flex the wrist so the fingers move toward the forearm. Keep the elbow straight. Turn the head to the opposite side, looking away from the wall for 10 repetitions. Repeat on the opposite side.

Figure 3.

90°/90° NERVE GLIDE

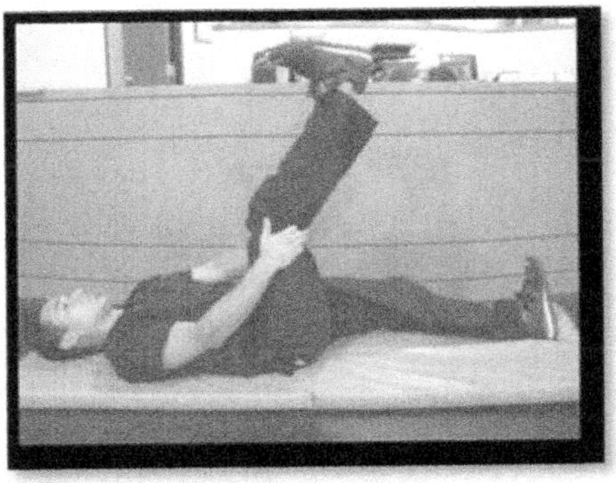

1. Lie on your back with one leg straight. Bring the opposite knee up towards chest so the hip and knee are bent to 90 degrees. Pull the foot and toes up like you are taking your foot off the gas pedal.

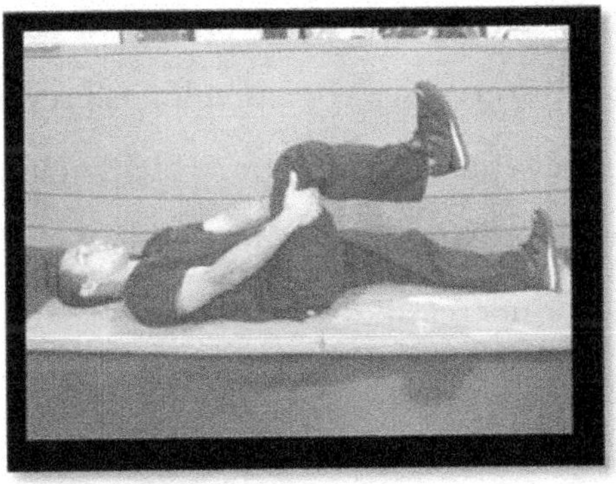

2. Keep the toes pointed up toward the nose. Extend the knee toward the sky. Stop when you pfeel a pull in the low back or anywhere along the leg.

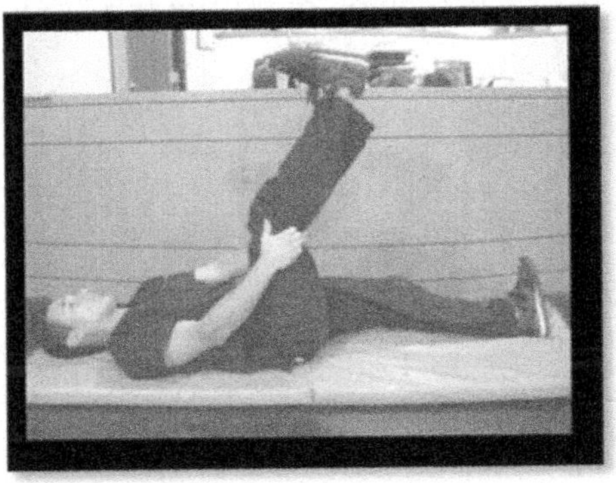

3. Relax the knee returning to the start position of 90 degrees of hip and knee flexion. Perform 10 repetitions. Repeat on the opposite leg.

Since the signal is unclear or reduced as it is sent to muscles in the legs, you may often feel a lack of control of the limbs. This can cause you to feel off balance. With regular exercise and balance training, you can improve the coordination of your legs to increase your safety and tolerance to walking, standing, climbing stairs, and recreational activity.

What if I have trouble with exercise?

Aquatic Therapy

We know you have pain. You are easily fatigued. Your bones may be weakened by the effects of multiple myeloma. Pool therapy provides a unique environment that can particularly benefit people with this disease as they transition into exercise. Therapeutic exercise performed in water utilizes the benefits of buoyancy, hydrostatic pressure, smooth resistance, temperature control, and variable depth to create an ideal environment for increasing strength safely and comfortably. You can learn the proper exercises and correct form in therapy with the intention of continuing aquatic exercises at your home, gym, or community pool. It can also help you in the transition from inactivity to land-based exercise.

Buoyancy

As the body is immersed in water, the property of buoyancy reduces the weight that is placed on the joints of the body. When you control the depth of the water you are exercising in, you can control the amount of weight that the body experiences. Thus, you can safely progress from a weakened state to an active lifestyle in a graduated manner. By limiting the amount of stress through the joints, healing is accelerated, tolerance to activity is enhanced, and outcomes are improved. Following fractures, the transition from a non-weight-bearing status to walking on land can be a painful and difficult experience. Utilizing the buoyancy of water supports the joints and reduces the stress to healing bones to create a smoother and faster transition to functional activities performed on land.

Hydrostatic Pressure

Swelling is a common part of the body's inflammatory response to tissue damage and injury. Whether it is the result of fractures, joint degeneration, circulatory problems, bed rest, poor posture, or an acute injury, swelling decreases the range of motion in the joints, ease of movement, and healing times. Swelling restricts the free flow of nutrient-rich blood to healing tissue. This slows or even prevents the body from healing. Multiple myeloma further reduces the body's ability to heal due to the reduction in the blood cell counts. The hydrostatic pressure of water creates compression to reduce and prevent swelling that may occur with exercise and injury.

Resistance

Smooth, non-impact resistance is created as the limbs are moved through water. As the velocity of movement increases, so does the resistance. This creates an infinite level of resistance with limitless adjustability to your level of fitness. Since we know your bones are weakened by multiple myeloma, high impact activities can result in fractures. The anemia associated with this condition can lead to bleeding and bruising. The water is a safe and supportive environment that allows you to perform the resisted activity necessary to build strength without the risk for fracture or excessive bleeding.

Temperature

Our pool is heated to 90 degrees to improve the flexibility of muscles and ligaments, ease movement, and increase circulation. The temperature of the pool can be manipulated to create an ideal environment for body movement. As tissue temperature increases, the extensibility and flexibility of muscles, ligaments, and tendons is enhanced. Greater extensibility reduces the joint's resistance to movement, making it feel more comfortable to exercise. When you take your program home, try to find a heated pool, or heat your pool if possible, to increase your tolerance to aquatic exercise.

Design

Our pool features variable depth including a deep-water well, underwater stairs, and resistance jets to create unique stations that stimulate healing, recovery and strengthening in a functional fashion. A hydraulic chair lift allows wheelchair-bound or severely deconditioned patients' access to our pool.

Variable Depth

The properties of compression and buoyancy are manipulated by varying the depth of submersion. The deep-water well is designed to allow for greater immersion in the water which substantially increases support to the body. Increased body support allows patients with poor balance, decreased postural support, restricted range of motion, and weakened muscles to perform therapeutic exercise in a safe and productive manner. Additionally, depth of submersion corresponds to the amount of compression to the joints. Compression can reduce and prevent swelling as well as provide external support to unstable joints.

Strength and coordination is a vital part of rehabilitation, recovery, and performance enhancement. Variation of depth creates a controllable amount of support for stretching and level of resistance for strengthening. Balance activities can be performed with changeable levels of support from the buoyancy of water to create a safe and comforting environment for patients with reduced postural stability. Even higher velocity activities performed in the water allow for the benefits of power movement with the safety and support of water.

Underwater Stairs

Stair negotiation training is augmented by the natural buoyancy of the body in water. We know weight bearing is important for building bone density, but you may not be able to tolerate standing on one leg with all of your weight. In order to go up and down stairs, you may need to build up to standing on one leg. Water provides a level of support to the body for patients unable to tolerate full weight bearing or lacking the strength and stability to lift their body weight without assistance when negotiating stairs. It is important that the joints of the hip, knee and ankle travel in the same plane when climbing stairs. This reduces the stress to the joint surface, the bones and the tendons that cross the joints. Physical therapists will show you how to perform exercise and functional stair negotiation in the best position possible.

Resistance Jets

In addition to resistance to movement through water, our pool allows for even greater control through resistance jets. Resistance jets create a turbulent flow of water that can be utilized to augment an endless number of therapeutic exercises and functional activities including specific upper and lower-extremity movement, walking, balance activities, and cardiovascular training. Furthermore, the resistance jets can be used for the massage of painful, sensitive areas when hands-on techniques may not be tolerated. If you have or have access to a hot tub, these jets can be used to control pain and muscle tension after you graduate from physical therapy.

What should I expect from Physical Therapy?

When you visit a physical therapist, you have an opportunity to have your questions answered. You can learn how to exercise correctly, what you should do to be active, and how you can continue to take care of yourself. You can attend therapy regularly or take what you learn home. It is up to you. Part of what we do is exercise-based, but it does not mean you have to pump iron. After an evaluation, your program will be tailored to your specific needs and goals. You will face challenges when starting an exercise program. You have pain and are tired. Your muscles may be weak. It may seem like a daunting task. With manual treatment, use of pain-relieving machines, thermal agents, and patient education, you can and will live a better life.

Success Stories

Mr. B

Dr. Berenson referred to us a 91-year-old man with multiple myeloma. He was a very successful businessman. At his initial evaluation, he complained of severe, debilitating low back pain after standing for longer than five minutes. This was a man who ran a very successful large corporation, but could not stand long enough to shave. He begrudgingly performed his exercises on the first visit. At first, his pain actually increased. He was sore, tired, and feeling helpless. He wanted to quit, but he kept coming in. After a couple of weeks, his wife started to notice he was standing up straighter. He began to report that he could stand for longer periods before the onset of his pain. He later told me that he had been able to attend a cocktail party without having to search for a chair as soon as he arrived. He was more active and regained his social life. The point is that it was not easy at first, but he didn't give up.

Mrs. M

Mrs. M was a very active 65-year-old cyclist and kayaker. She enjoyed kayaking out on the water with her husband, but fractures in her spine caused her to hunch over. She developed pain in both her shoulders as her posture deteriorated. It is a common problem for one complication to lead to another. By teaching her the correct position in which to hold her back and shoulder blades, she was able to restore her posture. She diligently performed her exercises and developed the endurance to maintain that posture when she returned to biking and paddling her kayak. You can be very active with multiple myeloma. You can even be active after the effects of the disease have taken their toll, but you have to work at it.

Any tips?

- Listen to your body. When you have pain or you are fatigued, you don't have to push it.
- Do what you can. Focus on the things you *can* do. Don't get discouraged by the things you can't do. You just may not be able to do them yet!

- Exercise at home. Exercise regularly. Stretching and exercise are more effective when performed consistently.
- Practice and improve your sleep position. What we do for a third of our lives can have a significant impact on how we feel when we are awake.
- Stand up straight, keep your knees and toes in line with each other, pull your shoulders back, and hold your head up. Posture is important for making us look and feel better.
- Worry only about the things you can control. You can increase your strength. You can improve your flexibility. You can fix your posture. You can live a better life.

You Have…

MULTIPLE MYELOMA!

WALDENSTROM'S MACROGLOBULINEMIA!

AMYLOIDOSIS!

MGUS!

(Monoclonal Gammopathy of Undetermined Significance)

By Jeffrey D. Waterman, DDS -- Periodontist

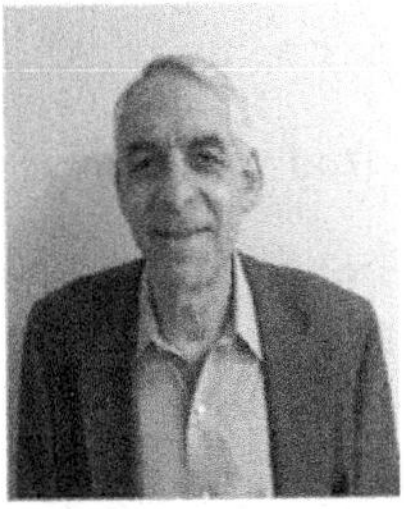

I am a periodontist by training. You may wonder why a dental specialist would be brought into the therapeutic loop in treating patients with multiple myeloma and other forms of metastatic forms of bone cancer. The reason is that the intravenous monthly bisphosphonate treatment (Aredia and Zometa), designed to strengthen the long bones of the body and to act directly on the cancer cells, and also has a potential serious side effect on the upper and/or lower jaw bones.

This side effect is known as osteonecrosis of the jaw or "ONJ." The symptoms of ONJ can include exposed bone with the loss of the soft tissue, as well as the spontaneous loss of teeth, infection and pain. The affected bone loses its cellularity and becomes brittle, essentially dead bone. The resulting infections can invade other structures including nerves, tissue spaces, and the sinuses. There is no cure for ONJ, but the vast majority of cases can be managed quite successfully. Our goal is to minimize or prevent ONJ. While this disease can occur spontaneously, in the absence of any associated dental causes, we know that it is very often associated with dental infections and dental surgery involving the jaw bone among patients receiving intravenously administered bisphosphonates. Dental extractions are perhaps the most common treatment often resulting in ONJ. While we make every effort to solve all pre-existing dental problems and avoid dental surgery prior to the initiation of bisphosphonate infusion therapy, it is sometimes necessary to proceed with surgical therapy even after the administration of the bisphosphonates has begun. It is recommended that a patient undergoes a complete dental examination (including head and neck) prior to beginning these monthly infusions. Any invasive dental procedures to solve these problems or to prevent the likelihood of serious problems occurring at a later date should be completed prior to the initiation of bisphosphonate therapy.

Dr. Berenson is one of the few oncologists, specializing in multiple myeloma, who recognizes the need for a referral for comprehensive dental evaluation prior to instituting bisphosphonate therapy. This evaluation should include a current set of full mouth X-rays as well as a panoramic X-ray, a complete medical history, including all current medications, diseases, allergies, and personal habits (smoking and or alcohol, recreational drugs, etc.). While the list of possible diagnostic areas to explore are too numerous to mention, special attention should be given to tumors and cysts of the jaws, impacted wisdom teeth, structurally weak or diseased teeth which may require fillings, crowns, root canals, extractions, periodontal surgery, dental implants, bridges, etc. Crowns and bridges on structurally weak teeth should not be undertaken. Any fractures or infections of the teeth into bone after bisphosphonate therapy has been initiated could put the patient at significant risk of developing ONJ. A full-mouth periodontal examination, including probing, tooth mobility, analysis of the bite, and evaluation of the soft tissues should also be performed.

In the area of prevention, many medications pose a risk of dry mouth, which is strongly associated with potential rampant tooth decay which ultimately increases the risk of ONJ if affected teeth require extraction. Thus, maintaining hydration is very important, but simply drinking more water does not work. There are special products such as Biotene and Oasis which offer artificial lubrication and can help to prevent dry mouth. Sometimes medications are associated with causing dry mouth but alternative medications are often not possible to prescribe. These especially include medications for the treatment of cardiovascular disease and pulmonary diseases. More recent research indicates that periodontal disease can exacerbate cardiovascular disease and diabetes.

All of this leads to another critical area of care which is the patient's personal responsibility in helping to prevent dental disease. Of course hard candy and foods high in refined sugar should be avoided. Oral hygiene is critical! This must include brushing (particularly at the gum line), flossing, and proxa-brushing. Dental disease is usually initiated between the teeth and using a toothbrush alone will not clean the areas between the teeth. The water pick is completely ineffective, as are mouthwashes. "Elbow grease" must be used, which, means flossing. The dentist must determine if the patient's dental hygiene is *effective*! If not, then instruction must be given and thorough professional dental cleanings should be done three to four times per year. Following completion of active dental therapy, it is often a good idea to be fitted for a bite splint (night guard). This will help to prevent the consequences of tooth grinding, leading to tooth fracture, which often occurs at night while sleeping. Teeth frequently fracture into the jaw bone, resulting in infection and necessitating surgical extraction (again possibly leading to ONJ).

What happens if ONJ is diagnosed after bisphosphonate therapy has already been administered? The most important action you can take is to see a competent dentist/surgeon who is well-informed regarding this disease. Extractions should be avoided at all costs unless there are no alternatives and it is absolutely necessary. I have developed a close relationship with an endodontist (a specialist in root canals) and we have been able to avoid, in most cases, removing what would have been considered hopeless teeth. Antimicrobial mouth rinses can be utilized, such as Peridex (chlorhexidine gluconate), bleach (20 parts water to one part bleach), and Betadine. Prominent, exposed bone spurs from ONJ can be reshaped and reduced without posing any threat to the patient. The use of antibiotics (often the use of two different antibiotics used concurrently) can be utilized effectively to control infection and pain; however, antibiotics should only be used for short-term therapy. Patients should not be kept on long-term antibiotics, as resistant strains of bacteria can develop and the antibiotics will then lose their effectiveness in treating dental or systemic infections in other areas of the body.

If dental extraction cannot be avoided, this should be handled by a competent, informed dental surgeon. First and foremost, a discussion must take place between the dental surgeon and the oncologist. If possible, a "drug holiday" should be initiated, waiting at least three months after ceasing bisphosphonate therapy before performing the extraction and for another three months after the procedure before restarting the treatment with Zometa or Aredia, although it is understood that sometimes this is not possible. Surgical techniques should be used to promote blood clot retention, maximizing the blood supply through the use of biologics, and surgical design to keep the jaw bone covered by soft tissue during healing. But again, I emphasize that one should avoid dental extractions and any invasive procedures involving the jaw bone whenever possible. All elective procedures such as periodontal surgery, dental implants, and risky restorative treatment should be avoided while patients are being treated with bisphosphonates.

The purpose of this chapter is to inform the patient that with preventive measures, proper diagnosis, self-care, and treatment, ONJ can often be prevented, or when it occurs, successfully managed. Early diagnosis and appropriate treatment are critical. Communication amongst specialists who are responsible for prevention, diagnosis, and management of ONJ, in concert with treatment of multiple myeloma and other forms of bone cancer, is critical. Lastly, having an informed patient who can understand this process and ask the right questions can often lead to the avoidance of critical mistakes by treating doctors.

You Have…

MULTIPLE MYELOMA!

WALDENSTROM'S MACROGLOBULINEMIA!

AMYLOIDOSIS!

MGUS!

(Monoclonal Gammopathy of Undetermined Significance)

By Laura Giffin Audell, MD -- Pain Specialist

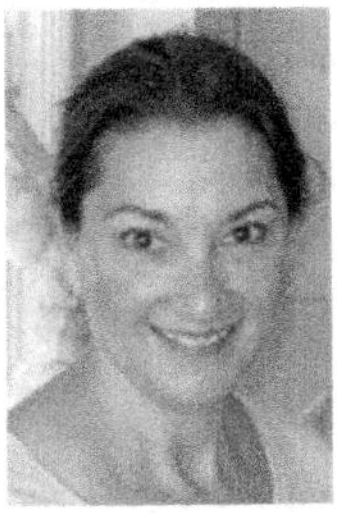

Pain is a cardinal presenting feature of myeloma, with pain being the problem that most often causes the patient to seek medical care. Pain can be insidious or acute, diffuse or localized with no one specific pattern. There is no classic presentation of the pain associated with myeloma. It can feel like a muscle ache, bone ache, nerve pain, or sudden severe musculoskeletal pain.

There are two general categories of pain that patients with myeloma experience: somatic and neuropathic pain. Somatic pain is pain due to tumor involvement of bone and associated structures, and neuropathic pain is due to nerve compression and irritation, or as a consequence of the effects of treatment on peripheral nerves.

Regardless of the type of pain, pain is worsened by poor sleep, fatigue, anxiety, depression, and stress. Each element of pain should be addressed to try to maximize quality of life and the ability to function. Sometimes treatment for one problem will also be the treatment for another. Treatment of the underlying myeloma is the most important treatment for pain in most cases, unless the cause of the pain is unrelated to the underlying cancer or from irreversible damage already done by the myeloma.

Somatic Pain

Treatment usually starts with the use of anti-inflammatory medications (aspirin-like drugs) if the patient does not have kidney involvement or poor kidney function. However, if they are taking steroids (e.g., dexamethasone, prednisone, or methylprednisolone), the combination of these types of drugs and anti-inflammatory agents increases the risk of gastrointestinal bleeding. Likewise, the use of acetaminophen (Tylenol) should be limited to no more than 2,000mg per day, so as not to stress the liver.

For mild to moderate pain, tramadol (Ultram) or tapentadol (Nucynta) may be helpful. If the patient is also on an antidepressant, the use of these drugs may be limited due to drug-drug interactions. The real possibility of drug-drug interactions is an excellent reason to get all of your medications from the same pharmacy. The computer programs in pharmacies will alert one to possible unwanted drug interactions.

Combination narcotic/acetaminophen medications such as hydrocodone/APAP (Vicodin, Norco, Lortab or Lorcet) or oxycodone/APAP (Percocet, Endocet) can be used, with the daily dose limited largely because of the amount of acetaminophen (Tylenol) in these combination medications. Higher doses of the hydrocodone combinations are also not desirable due to the potential permanent neurosensory (nerve-related) hearing loss. Higher doses of oxycodone can be used without the added acetaminophen using oxycodone tablets in different strengths and/or the sustained release form of oxycodone.

There are other narcotic analgesics that can be adjusted as needed to control pain, but the need for pain relief must be balanced against the potential sedating (sleepiness) and constipating side effects of the narcotics. Often patients do best with a low dose of sustained-release medications along with a shorter acting medication with a rapid onset of action, which is used on an as-needed basis if the patient experiences acute onset of pain or will be participating in activities that are likely to bring on pain.

Narcotic medications should be reduced to the lowest effective dose whenever possible to prevent the onset of tolerance and other side effects such as somnolence. Tolerance occurs when a patient has been using narcotics on a regular basis. It is more frequently seen with higher doses of these medications. Over time, the patient may require higher and higher doses of medication to achieve the same reduction in pain. When this occurs, a rotation to another regime of medication is often in order, especially if clinically there has been no change in the patient's condition.

If a patient is experiencing pain from a fracture, calcitonin may be helpful. Calcitonin is a bone hormone that decreases bone pain probably through a mechanism involving a neurotransmitter of pain. Calcitonin is usually used for this purpose for one to two months only. Intravenous monthly infusions of zoledronic acid (Zometa) or pamidronate (Aredia) have also been shown to help relieve bone pin. Lidocaine patches may also be prescribed to be used in the area of pain from vertebral or spinal compression fractures. They work by locally numbing the area of ache. Transcutaneous electrical nerve stimulators (TENS) units can be used to give counter stimulation in areas of hurt. The brain pays attention to the buzzing sensation from the TENS unit, and not to the underlying ache. There is also an increase in endorphins released locally from the TENS stimulation which also helps pain.

Patients will often experience significant muscle spasm associated with vertebral fractures. Very frequently, the pain from the spasm can be as bad as or even worse than the fracture itself, and involve a larger area of the back. Spasm pain is poorly treated with narcotics. If the pain is mostly spasm, a muscle relaxant is the best treatment. There are several different kinds of muscle relaxants, so it may take a bit of trial and error to find one that is effective and does not cause the patient to feel too drowsy.

Complementary treatments for pain can include gentle massage, gentle physical therapy, gentle stretching with an emphasis on posture, and balance training. Pool or water therapy to help with rehabilitation can help a patient recover from fracture and its associated muscle spasms. Some patients will benefit from "balancing" acupuncture. A healthy diet cannot be underestimated in helping a person feel better. Adequate sleep is very important, taking short naps when needed, but not after 3:00 p.m. so as not to interfere with the normal sleep cycle.

Neuropathic Pain

Sometimes the source of pain is from the nerves themselves. Myeloma can interfere with nerve function, as can the medications used to treat the disease. This will often manifest itself as a peripheral neuropathy, with numbness, tingling, and burning pain in the hands and feet. Alpha-lipoic acid, a dietary supplement, is often given to myeloma patients to try to prevent the onset of neuropathy. The usual dose is 600mg per day up to 1,800mg per day. Sometimes, prescription B complex vitamins (Metanx) will also be given to try to prevent onset of neuropathy. It is also important to maintain vitamin D levels in the normal range. Some studies in other diseases such as diabetes have shown that those with low vitamin D levels have a higher risk of peripheral neuropathy.

The mainstays of treatment for neuropathic pain, once it occurs, is usually a combination of membrane-stabilizing medications such as gabapentin (Neurontin) or pregabalin (Lyrica), and antidepressants in the SNRI class of medications such as duloxitene (Cymbalta) and venlafaxine (Effexor). Many antidepressants have no effect on pain. Medications in the SSRI class, such as fluoxetine (Prozac), citalopram HBr (Celexa), and paroxetine hydrochloride (Paxil) have no effect on pain, although they can be very effective antidepressants. Membrane stabilizing medications work by decreasing the irritability of damaged nerves, and thus make them less likely to spontaneously fire and send painful messages. The antidepressants have direct effects also on the nerves, but also change the attention paid to the pain at the level of the brain. Some of the older antidepressants can be very helpful for neuropathic pain, and help with normal REM sleep. These include amitriptyline (Elavil), nortriptyline (Pamelor), and doxepin (Sinequan). These medications are generally much less expensive, but their use is limited by side effects of dry mouth, constipation, and orthostatic hypotension, or decreased blood pressure with standing.

Other Important Considerations

Regardless of the type of pain, somatic or neuropathic, the effect on the person can be lessened by improving quality of sleep, decreasing depression, and especially decreasing anxiety. Maintaining normal sleep-wake cycles is very important. Spending at least 20 minutes outside on a daily basis is important to a normal circadian rhythm. Light exercise, such as daily walking for 20 minutes, helps with bone and muscle strength. Daily exercise also helps with sleep quality.

Depression frequently occurs in persons facing life-threatening illnesses. Acknowledging it and treating it with medication or therapy is very helpful in getting a person through their myeloma-related problems and side effects from its treatment. It will also lessen the effect it can have on the pain. Untreated depression can worsen pain, and increase the suffering that pain can bring on. Suffering can be lessened through cognitive behavioral techniques, as can anxiety.

Perhaps the condition that has the largest impact on pain is anxiety. Anxiety causes release of the fight and flight neurotransmitters, epinephrine and norepinephrine. This is what causes the rapid heartbeat, sweating, and irritability that come with anxiety. Epinephrine and norepinephrine also function as neurotransmitters of pain. They are part of the chemical relay system that transmits the pain impulse to the brain. Anxiolytics, medications designed specifically for the treatment of anxiety can help. These medications include lorazepam (Ativan), clonazepam (Klonopin), and alprazolam

(Xanax). Another excellent treatment for anxiety can be Cognitive Behavioral Therapy (CBT). The person learns through skill training usually with a psychologist trained in CBT to recognize and stop anxiety symptoms before they take on a life of their own. Once learned, these skills can be used for any variety of symptoms. This is not hocus pocus. These techniques are learned and employed by the US Navy Seals.

Finally, being able to continue to engage in those things that make you happy while you are going through your treatment remains an important goal of pain management. The purpose of pain management is to not only to treat the pain itself, but to help maintain the quality of life while undergoing lifesaving treatment.

You Have…

MULTIPLE MYELOMA!

WALDENSTROM'S MACROGLOBULINEMIA!

AMYLOIDOSIS!

MGUS!

(Monoclonal Gammopathy of Undetermined Significance)

By Mary Donkersloot, RD – Nutritionist

Smart Eating Show on Instagram, Facebook, YouTube

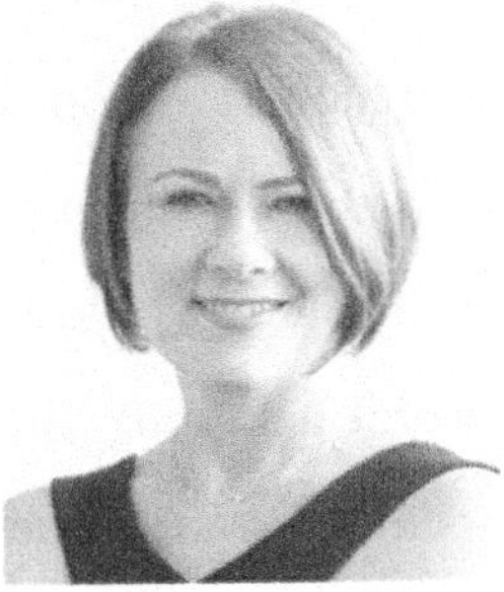

When you have multiple myeloma, there are a few nutritional issues you may need to address, and this chapter is an encapsulation of those concerns.

In general terms, there is limited research on a diet that can decrease or treat the disease or help reduce the side effects from the treatment. Anecdotal reports on the Internet make claims that a diet low in sugar, saturated fat, and alcohol but with lots of fruits and vegetables can help patients achieve remissions. This is also known as an anti-inflammatory diet, and I try to eat that way myself. It is the best diet to avoid a host of issues, including heart disease, autoimmune issues, and some kinds of cancers, even if there is no direct evidence of its effects on multiple myeloma. For the record, multiple myeloma is not an autoimmune disease.

Regardless, a clean diet just makes good common sense. Avoiding "fake" foods with lots of additives and preservatives and artificial sweeteners is important for all patients. Try to keep packaged foods like baked goods to a limit. For example, if you must eat a protein bar or ice cream, look for one with five ingredients or less. Skip soda or diet soda and instead drink water, tea, or coffee.

That said, there are a few nutritional issues specific to multiple myeloma:

Hypercalcemia: This is the most common metabolic complication of multiple myeloma. When bone cells break down, which commonly occurs in myeloma patients, calcium can leach from the bones into the blood and create dangerously high levels of calcium in the blood. Your doctor will treat this with drugs such as zoledronic acid, but you also need to stop taking your calcium supplements and avoid foods high in calcium. In addition, remember that vitamin D helps bring calcium into the body through the gastrointestinal tract, so stop taking it if your calcium is too high. Your doctor is likely to give you intravenous fluids containing sodium. Consequently, you may also benefit by being a bit more liberal with the salt-shaker since sodium can liberate calcium into the urine. It's ironic, since we hear so much about Americans eating too much salt, but in this circumstance, salt may be your friend if your calcium is too high.

Magnesium: Some people with multiple myeloma have low magnesium levels from poor nutrition. Magnesium along with vitamin D helps regulate calcium levels and can help strengthen bone. If you don't have high calcium in your blood, supplement your diet with 1 gram of magnesium per day. Magnesium may also help with peripheral neuropathy. By the way, so can alpha lipoic acid—600 mg daily. Magnesium can also help with constipation that can result from chemo drugs, but too much can cause diarrhea. Once your doctor checks your levels, you can determine the level of supplement that may help you, but 250 mg twice daily is a common dose. Green leafy vegetables, nuts, and halibut are all good sources of magnesium.

Vitamin D: One quarter to one third of people with multiple myeloma are vitamin D deficient. Dr. Berenson has been studying vitamin D, which works with calcium to help build healthy bones and reduces the risk of bone-related complications such as fracture. It also has an impact on the heart and immune system. The effects of vitamin D are far-reaching and some studies show keeping the levels in the right ranges may also help decrease weakness, fatigue, and the severity of peripheral neuropathy (numbness, tingling, and sometimes pain in the hands and feet).

It is a good idea to have your vitamin D level checked and aim for a level of at least 30. Some research shows that a level of closer to 50 or even 70 may provide health benefits and decrease pain. Depending on your level, you may want to take a supplement.

If your level is low, you should start with a higher weekly dose—usually 50,000 IU once weekly, which can be taken orally. Once you get to a level above at least 30, you can usually keep your level there with 1000–2000 IU per day, but you may require additional supplementation, especially if you are trying to keep your levels higher (50–70). Dietary sources of vitamin D include dairy products as well as alternatives like fortified soy milk, almond milk, and rice milk, which are generally fortified with vitamin D as well as calcium. Fatty fish is also a good source of vitamin D, and you get the bonus of omega three fatty acids as well. And don't forget sun exposure, a great way to keep levels in a protective range.

Iron: Anemia is a low red blood cell count and is a common problem for multiple myeloma patients. Since red blood cells are produced in the bone marrow, which can be filled with myeloma tumor cells, this disease can result in suppression of production of red blood cells, which is anemia. Red blood cells transport oxygen to the tissues, and when levels are low, exhaustion and fatigue occur. However, many patients actually have other causes for their low red blood cell counts, such as low iron or vitamin B12 levels. If these are the causes, supplements of these products may reverse the anemia. In addition, excellent sources of dietary iron include red meat, pork, chicken, beans, legumes, leafy greens (especially spinach), dried fruit, and iron-fortified grains. If one has low iron levels, it is important to look for a cause, which is often due to a loss of blood in the gastrointestinal tract. High levels of vitamin B12 are found in meat, salmon, cod, dairy products, eggs, and fortified grains.

Vitamin C: Perhaps the most highly researched nutrient related to cancer, vitamin C helps protect cells from free radical damage that may lead to cancer. This is likely one of many reasons why a diet high in fruits and vegetables protects us from so many disease states. It is best to get your vitamin C from plenty of fruits and vegetables, since these contain an abundance of many other nutrients as well, and isolating this vitamin doesn't make sense when you have so many other nutritional benefits from these foods, many of which are yet to be discovered!

(Note: If you're taking bortezomib, be aware that vitamin C degrades this drug and reduces its therapeutic effect, so avoiding its use within several hours of receiving bortezomib is important. Regular intake of fruits and vegetables are fine, just not in higher doses that would come in pill form.)

It is also possible that vitamin C can improve the effectiveness of some chemotherapy agents commonly used to treat multiple myeloma, such as melphalan and cyclophosphamide, through its effects to increase free radical levels in cancer cells.

Protein: Protein not only helps the body repair cells and build muscle tissue, but it also supports the recovery of the immune system. Keep protein levels high enough to maintain muscle mass and strength. A malnourished state leads to a low albumin level which causes edema (swelling), most commonly in the ankles and feet. There may be times when you have nausea or loss of appetite, and consequently eat less and lose weight. With an adequate protein in your diet of about 20–30 grams, 3–4 times per day, you will be more likely to maintain your strength, as long as your calorie intake is also adequate. A piece of fish or chicken the size of the palm of your hand is about four ounces and 30 grams of protein. You don't need more than that at one meal, since your body can't assimilate that much at one time. Good sources of protein include eggs, dairy products, nuts, beans, and tofu.

Sugar: If you're on steroids, you may do well to limit sugar and high glycemic carbs like pasta, white rice, white bread, and desserts, which contain high levels of sugar. Insulin is a hormone made by the pancreas that increases after you eat in order to move the sugar from the blood into the cells. Steroids can make it hard for cells in your body to use insulin, which leads to high blood sugar levels. So, if you're on a steroid, go easy on sugar and high glycemic foods.

(Note: The addition of the antibiotic clarithromycin, which is often used for treating multiple myeloma can increase the side effects of steroids and raise blood sugar levels further. So, it is important to monitor your blood sugar closely when you are taking this antibiotic with steroids.)

Water: Staying hydrated helps to protect your kidney function as well as flush the drugs that are used to treat the myeloma out of your system. Maintain a strong hydration status by starting with fluids early in the day, two liters a day for women, and three for men. A good test is relatively clear urine, or at least urine that is not too concentrated. By the way, water, coffee, and tea do count, but it is good to avoid sugary beverages. Be careful to not drink a lot of only water, as this can lower your sodium, so liquids containing electrolytes can help with this. Keep a liter bottle or carafe of water or liquids by your side throughout the day so you can monitor your intake to make sure you reach your target. You may have to make frequent trips to the bathroom, but the benefits are well worth it!

By now you are beginning to understand that diet plays a very important role in managing multiple myeloma. This chapter touches on only a few of the issues. For more information, and for a personal nutrition plan, ask your doctor for a referral to a Registered Dietitian Nutritionist who is informed about multiple myeloma.

You Have…

MULTIPLE MYELOMA!

WALDENSTROM'S MACROGLOBULINEMIA!

AMYLOIDOSIS!

MGUS!

(Monoclonal Gammopathy of Undetermined Significance)

By Michael Levine, MD -- Nephrologist

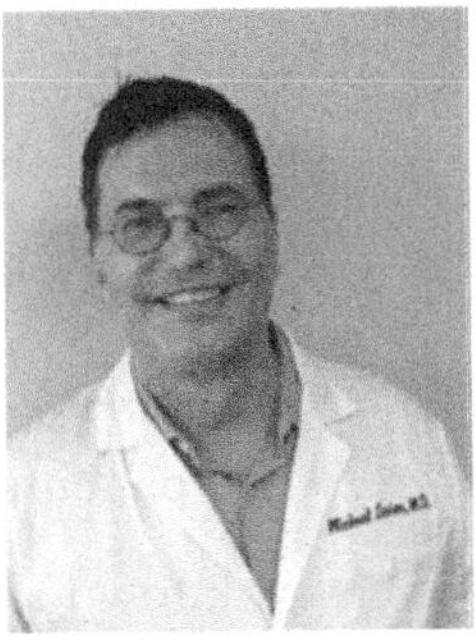

When I tell people that I'm a nephrologist, I usually add "a kidney doctor," as I often see a puzzled look if I don't. Myeloma frequently affects the kidneys. Often the nephrologist is the first doctor to diagnose myeloma, as kidney involvement in myeloma can be the presenting manifestation of the disease.

Myeloma can injure the kidneys in a number of ways, but the most common involves the deposition of a type of protein ("light chain") in the kidney that causes damage. Some myeloma patients accumulate an abnormal protein called amyloid, and this can also cause kidney damage. Patients with high uric acid levels can also have kidney injury, often with aggressive disease or after chemotherapy.

The main function of the kidneys is to excrete excess fluid, minerals such as sodium and potassium, and wastes including blood urea nitrogen (BUN) and creatinine. When I see a patient with myeloma and kidney disease, I always ask if they know their creatinine level. Creatinine is a toxin that is normally excreted by the kidneys, and a normal level for most laboratories is less than 1.2. Patients with poor kidney function or on dialysis often have very high creatinine levels, in the range of 5–10. Often the creatinine level is the best test to follow to determine the level of kidney function. It's common to see improvement in the creatinine level with a response to the myeloma treatment with the effective therapies now available to patients. Lowering the myeloma cell numbers with effective therapy will result in a reduction in the light chains. This can lead to significant and at times dramatic improvement in renal function for patients with kidney disease due to myeloma.

Sometimes myeloma leads to severe kidney disease, and patients develop symptoms of loss of appetite, nausea, and lethargy, known as uremia. Dialysis is performed if these symptoms develop. Hemodialysis involves cleaning the blood with the artificial kidney machine. Typically, hemodialysis is given three times per week for several hours at a time. Another kind of dialysis is peritoneal dialysis, which involves placement of a tube in the abdomen. This type of dialysis is performed at home by the patient, often at night during sleep using a special peritoneal dialysis machine. Fluid goes in and out of the abdominal cavity and wastes are removed.

It is important to note that patients with myeloma requiring dialysis can often regain enough renal function with effective treatment that they no longer require this procedure, so its use is not always permanent. Today, patients with myeloma rarely remain on chronic dialysis.

There are measures that improve kidney function in myeloma patients in addition to chemotherapy. Hydration and the use of alkali (bicarbonate) can increase the solubility of the light chains so they are no longer toxic, and, thus, prevent kidney damage. It is important to avoid drugs that can decrease kidney function, including anti-inflammatory drugs such as ibuprofen. Low protein diets can decrease symptoms of kidney failure and may prevent the progression of renal disease. Restriction of fluid, salt, and potassium is sometimes needed. Kidney patients can develop bone disease, particularly if they have myeloma. Many myeloma patients have low vitamin D levels and often supplemental vitamin D is given to prevent bone pain and fractures.

You Have…

MULTIPLE MYELOMA!

WALDENSTROM'S MACROGLOBULINEMIA!

AMYLOIDOSIS!

MGUS!

(Monoclonal Gammopathy of Undetermined Significance)

By Regina Swift, RN – Myeloma Specialist
Berenson Oncology

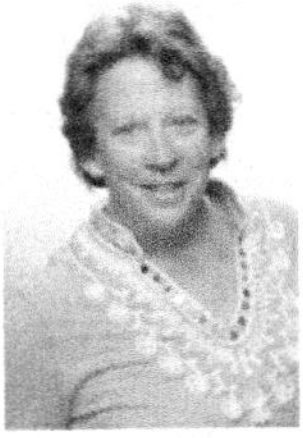

The answer is multiple myeloma. No, it's not melanoma, it is myeloma! "Am I going to die?" "Will I ever feel normal again?" "I can't take the pain, I can't walk very far, I am so tired." The questions are never ending. Where to begin?

It is easy to understand why patients get easily confused. The two diseases begin with "M" and end in "oma." However, they are different. Melanoma is a cancer of the skin and is more recognized than myeloma. Myeloma is a cancer of the bone marrow, specifically of a type of white blood cell called a plasma cell. Now that we have clarified that myeloma and melanoma are different diseases, we can begin to address other issues.

To address the other questions, we need to be patient-specific. The one lesson I have learned from Dr. Berenson, in the 20 years that we have worked together, is that if we don't treat and get the disease under control for the patients that require therapy, you will never see improvement in how the patient feels. This concept is so true! However, for a nurse who likes to take the road with fewer bumps, this can be a very scary ride.

As clinicians, treating a patient who is already in a precarious predicament, with lab values that already are poor because of their disease state and often worsen with treatment, can be a daunting task. It feels as though we walk a very fine line. It probably took me easily three years, before I eased up on feeling so uncomfortable with this journey. I say "eased up" because I still get quite harried at times as I deal with the many nuances of taking care of this complex disease. There are many hurdles that have to be overcome so that our patients can enjoy the best and longest lives possible. However, I began to learn the patterns. What can I do to be proactive? Maybe you should come in on Friday and we check your labs again? This way if you need blood or platelets you can get them so there are no problems over the weekend. This is just one of many practical issues that have come up with our patients over many years.

Patients who present with their disease being the most active are usually the very sickest. Treatment needs to begin sooner than later. Patients sometimes think they can start treatment and then one month later take a vacation, but this does not allow us to give them the best chance to get the disease under control. In general, a minimum of three cycles (usually months) is needed before we know if the treatment has been successful. What is the definition of successful? First and foremost, it means the myeloma numbers decrease or, as in many cases today, disappear altogether. However, this usually does not mean that the disease is gone forever.

Numbers… what numbers are we talking about? This is an entirely separate educational session. Briefly, there are three specific markers we routinely follow in myeloma patients, including the serum monoclonal protein level, amount of 24-hour urine monoclonal protein, and serum free light chain level. We routinely monitor all three of these markers on a monthly basis, which gives us our best chance of accurately following the patient's response to their treatment. Markers are the numerical or quantifiable ways that we monitor improvement or progression (worsening) of the patient's disease. However, we must also observe and listen to the patient, because sometimes symptoms appear that tell us the patient's disease is getting worse before the markers do.

One of my greatest frustrations in dealing with myeloma is that there are generic aspects of the disease (i.e., bone involvement, anemia, thrombocytopenia [low platelet count], etc.), yet the degree or severity of each of these complications is patient-specific. No one treatment works for every patient. Nor are the side effects of a specific treatment the same for every patient. If I could ask one thing of all the patients in our clinic, it would be to remember those two points.

Our patients believe in being informed and educated about their disease, but sometimes in their sharing, they forget that just because they reacted poorly to a treatment, does not mean that the person they are talking to will react in the same way, both in terms of their ability to tolerate the treatment as well as the response of their disease to it. However, after conversations with other patients, some become averse to trying a therapy they have not been treated with because of what they have heard from other patients. So please continue to share your experiences with others, but remember to perhaps filter the negatives so you don't put another patient at risk of never getting what may turn out to be both a highly effective and well-tolerated treatment.

My other frustration is the randomness of it all. Why do some patients have disease that is very responsive and others have disease that is just so resistant or aggressive. I have come to accept that I will probably never have an answer for this, but I will never stop asking why.

Will there ever be cure for myeloma? I certainly hope so! I believe that the work of doctors such as James Berenson and the Institute for Myeloma & Bone Cancer Research (IMBCR) has led the charge in that direction. However, that goal of finding a cure takes time and financial resources. So I hope the generosity we have received already to support the research will continue and grow in the future.

I also believe that the patients who have participated in the many clinical trials we have conducted over the years have been key players in the discovery of new effective and well-tolerated therapies that are now used all over the world to treat myeloma and related diseases. Thank you to our patients for helping yourselves and future myeloma patients.

Over the past two decades we have seen such growth in the field of drug discovery for the treatment of myeloma. Thanks to Dr. Berenson and his clinical trials, we have been there from the ground floor in the development of these new effective therapies. It is rewarding to see a drug go from the lab to trial development and then finally to FDA approval! It is also so rewarding to then have an extremely sick patient, give them one of these ground breaking treatments, and within one or two months see a completely different person who is back to the activities that he or she enjoyed before they became ill.

I truly am blessed to have come in contact with Dr. Berenson, to enjoy the work that I do, to have forged friendships with many of the patients, and to have them still here 20 years later. If the cure is not in sight, then let us treat this disease as a chronic illness that we can manage with the best outcomes until the cure arrives, hopefully in the not too distant future.

"A Good Beginning is Half the Work"

You Have…

MULTIPLE MYELOMA!

WALDENSTROM'S MACROGLOBULINEMIA!

AMYLOIDOSIS!

MGUS!

(Monoclonal Gammopathy of Undetermined Significance)

By Richard T. Sokolov, MD -- Infectious Diseases

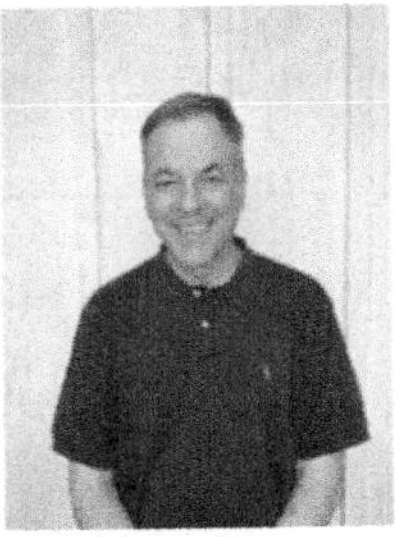

Immunoglobulins, or antibodies, are complex proteins that are critical in providing our defense against infections. We are exposed to a wide variety of infectious organisms, and the body normally produces many different types of antibodies to deal with this vast array. These infections are mostly due to bacteria that possess a capsule on their surface but also can involve infections from fungal organisms and viruses.

Multiple myeloma is a malignancy involving a type of cell known as a plasma cell, which makes antibodies. Patients with multiple myeloma and related disorders produce large amounts of antibodies as a result of the overabundance of plasma cells in their body. Unfortunately, the antibodies produced by the plasma cells in each patient are all of the same type, and these patients lack the vast array of other antibodies necessary to fend off the many infectious organisms that they contact. For this reason, infection is a major cause of morbidity and mortality in multiple myeloma.

It is the responsibility of the hematologist or oncologist, and in some cases infectious disease physicians, to prevent and recognize these infections before they become a major problem for these patients. Thus, early recognition is the key to survival in many cases.

Many different types of organisms can be involved in infections in multiple myeloma patients. However, one organism stands out. That is the pneumococcus. This particular bacterium poses a very significant threat to patients with multiple myeloma and related disorders. This is because the pneumococcus has a thick capsule around it (almost like a jacket) that allows it to elude and evade the immune system unless very specific antibodies are present to fight them.

There are multiple different sites in the body where infection can occur in MM patients. Specific infections include those of the lungs (pneumonias), skin and soft tissue infections anywhere in the body, urinary tract infections, and even meningitis (an infection in the fluid compartment that surrounds and cushions the brain and the spinal cord).

Multiple myeloma patients require early aggressive use of antibiotics (anti-infective medications) at the very first sign of an infection.

Early clues to the presence of infections may include the following:

1. Fevers
2. Sweats
3. Chills
4. Cough
5. Headaches
6. Shortness of breath
7. Rhinorrhea (runny nose)
8. Dysuria (pain on urination)
9. Rash
10. Redness, swelling, and pain in the skin
11. Pain in the bone or joint

Patients with multiple myeloma frequently need large, chronic indwelling catheters in their chest or extremities. These go by the name of "ports" or "PICC-lines". These devices allow patients to receive frequent infusions for their treatments and blood draws without having to be stuck with a needle every time such services are necessary. While these port catheters and PICC lines can improve the quality of life for multiple myeloma patients, they themselves may be sites of infection and may place the patient at an increased risk. This is because these devices create small defects in the skin through which bacteria may gain access to the body and spread quickly.

The chemotherapy itself may also predispose or increase the risk of infections in myeloma patients. The chemotherapy targets and destroys rapidly dividing cells, especially the tumor cells. However, the chemotherapy can also affect the patient's white blood cells, especially the neutrophils, which are also critical in fighting infection. Because these cells (like immunoglobulins) are critical in fighting infections and their levels often fall in response to chemotherapy, patients receiving this type of treatment are at high risk of developing infections.

In addition to lowering the white blood cell count, some of the drugs used for the treatment of multiple myeloma may also cause unique immune defects that may increase susceptibility to viral infections, especially a virus called "varicella." This virus is the cause of childhood chicken pox and zoster (or shingles) in adults. The latter is a very painful cutaneous eruption that can cause chronic suffering and at times can even disseminate and threaten patient's lives.

There exist several strategies for myeloma patients to minimize their risk of developing infectious disease complications. Early initiation of anti-infective therapy is critical when indicated. Antibiotics are used based on the specific organism that is causing the infection, and in some cases more than one antibiotic may have to be used. Although antibiotics may help fight off the infection, sometimes these drugs may predispose the patient to additional infections involving organisms such as various fungi and *Clostridia difficile*, which may cause protracted diarrhea.

Because multiple myeloma patients are at risk of kidney damage from their disease, the antibiotics employed are principally those that are least likely to cause kidney insufficiency or direct injury to the kidneys. In addition, some of the drugs may be broken down in the kidney so that with impaired kidney function, the dose of these agents may have to be reduced.

In addition to starting antimicrobials early, preemptive vaccination against infections that myeloma patients are uniquely susceptible to can be critical. The most important here would be vaccines against pneumococcus and seasonal influenza (flu) viruses. A vaccine exists against varicella but it is not recommended for myeloma patients since it is a live virus vaccine and myeloma patients have an impaired ability to deal with viral infections from their underlying immune deficient state. Moreover, although vaccination against pneumococcus and flu is recommended, the effectiveness of these vaccines is more limited in myeloma patients because of their impaired immune state.

Meticulous care of the chronic indwelling catheters is also important. Patient's families, nurses, and physicians must be vigilant to the conditions of these catheters and keep these sites clean at all times.

When the white blood cell count falls too low due to chemotherapy, there are drugs that can increase the white blood cell count. One such drug is granulocyte-colony stimulating factor (G-CSF), which can be given as Neupogen or Neulasta. This agent can elevate the white blood cells quickly when the white blood cells are depressed as a result of chemotherapy and help reduce the patient's risk of infection.

Patient education regarding the early signs and symptoms of infection and also informing family and caregivers can be critical towards early institution of therapy and recognition of infections.

Patients and families are also told to avoid other ill patients or crowded congested situations where myeloma may have close contact with potentially ill patients.

This includes:

1. Avoid children with cough, colds, or diarrhea.
2. Avoid crowded places like churches, temples, sporting events, and movie theaters.
3. And it is critical to keep the caregivers in good health.

Influenza in a healthy caregiver may be a nuisance illness for several days, but if the caregiver was to give influenza to a multiple myeloma patient, the complication could be disastrous and even life-threatening.

Finally, caregivers must employ meticulous hygiene when in close contact with patients, particularly hand hygiene with a chlorhexidine-containing product.

With proper preventative measures and quick intervention when infection strikes a myeloma patient, the effects of these complications can be minimized.

You Have…

MULTIPLE MYELOMA!

WALDENSTROM'S MACROGLOBULINEMIA!

AMYLOIDOSIS!

MGUS!

(Monoclonal Gammopathy of Undetermined Significance)

By Robert A. Audell, MD -- Orthopedist

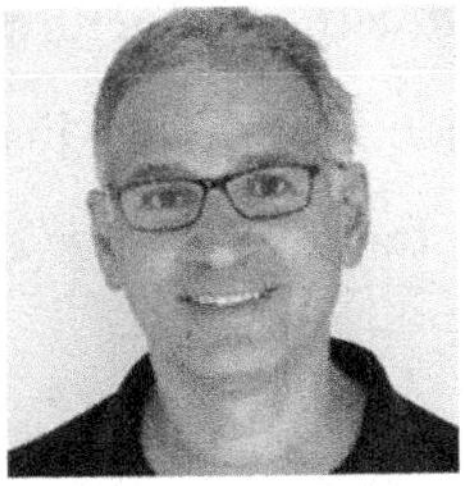

Multiple myeloma is the most common bone cancer that arises directly from bone tissue. The cell type responsible for myeloma is the *plasma cell,* which resides in the area of bone that makes blood and its components, the *bone marrow*. It manifests itself in many ways both obvious and occult. Surprisingly, perhaps, the most serious effects of the disease do not affect the bone at all, but other organs such as the kidneys. Nevertheless, bone problems occur in almost everyone who has this condition and remain the major clinical manifestation of the disease. These problems present special challenges for those who care for myeloma patients.

The most common effects of myeloma on bone are *fractures* (broken bones) resulting from complex biochemical processes that weaken the bone both locally, at the site of a collection of plasma cells, and generally, by depleting all bones of calcium and its associated bone matrix. The result of these fractures is pain, deformity, and rarely paralysis. Since myeloma affects the bone marrow, fractures usually occur in the bone that is part of the marrow or next to it. These areas are the skull, spine, shoulder blades, ribs, pelvis, shoulders, and hips. Fractures outside of the "center" of the body (*axial skeleton*) are uncommon.

Orthopedic intervention in the patient with multiple myeloma is directed at treating and preventing the effects of the broken bones. Bone pain is present in myeloma patients with and without fractures but, in general, patients experience worse pain when a bone has just fractured or is extremely weakened and ready to fracture (*impending fracture*).

There are multiple strategies that physicians use to address the problems of fractures in myeloma patients. It cannot be stressed enough that the primary method to prevent and treat bone problems is effective intervention by the patient's oncologist to deal with the patient's myeloma with treatment strategies that reduce the burden of multiple myeloma. All other care is secondary both in urgency and importance. In most cases, care should be directed at bone-related issues with surgery, and radiation therapy should occur after the myeloma treatment has begun to control the underlying disease. However, sometimes immediate attention must be given to the patient's bone-related problems, especially with significant fractures that require immediate repair, unstable spine conditions, or when the spinal cord is being compressed by the myeloma.

Orthopedists approach fracture treatment in the presence of myeloma and other medical conditions in a similar manner. A fracture is realigned and then supported. Typically, in a normal individual with, for example, a wrist fracture, the bone is manipulated back to normal alignment and then held in that position with a cast. If the orthopedist, based on experience, knows that a particular fracture will tend to lose alignment with simple casting, then a decision is made to stabilize the broken bone surgically. In the specific case of spinal fractures, realignment is often achieved by careful positioning on a fracture table and normal bone fixation is achieved using screws and rods or other metallic devices.

Fortunately for both the patient and physician, myeloma bone fractures tend to heal quickly with proper management often with a concomitant significant and rapid reduction in bone pain.

The fixation chosen depends on many factors, including the location of the fracture, the severity of the fracture, and the strength of the bone. The last factor is of particular importance in the myeloma patient. When the bone is very soft, as is the case in myeloma, many types of fixation will fail by pulling out of the bone. Often this means that fixation with metal implants is of limited utility and additional fixation using bone cement (poly methyl methacrylate or PMMA) is necessary.

In my practice, I am most commonly asked to treat spinal fractures of the mid and low back in myeloma patients. These fractures are remote and traditionally have been difficult to realign and fix without a large open surgery using metallic fixation devices. As a result, until about 10 years ago most patients presenting with spine fractures were given *radiation therapy* to treat the local plasma cell collection. While this intervention is undeniably helpful in removing local tumor collections, it unfortunately does not address the collapse and deformity associated with spine fractures nor does it adequately treat pain in many patients as well as the remainder of the disease elsewhere. Radiation treatment can also cause significant side effects, compromising the bone marrow function and preventing the use of effective drugs to treat the myeloma, and delaying the start of therapy required to treat the myeloma present throughout the bone marrow. In addition, several effective myeloma drugs increase the side effects of radiation therapy, which may prevent their use if radiation therapy is given.

In early 2002, based on my frustration with then-available treatment options for myeloma patients presenting with spine fractures and back pain, I began to perform balloon kyphoplasties to realign and fix spinal fractures in the mid and low back. The procedure often resulted in immediate and lasting pain relief with minimal risks. Pre-operative evaluation usually requires magnetic imaging (MRI) or computed tomography (CAT) to better delineate the nature and extent of tumor involvement in the involved areas in the spine. The kyphoplasty procedure itself is performed using X-ray guidance through small incisions in a procedure or operating room. This technique involves use of a needle that is placed at the site of the fracture with a balloon that is expanded, creating a cavity in which cement is placed to regain vertebral body height and stabilize the fracture. Complications can occur, but it is generally extremely safe in experienced hands and certainly has fewer problems than the more invasive older procedures. In most circumstances, kyphoplasty is performed in the hospital with at most an overnight stay. Now this procedure has largely become the standard of care for treating vertebral compression fractures in cancer patients, including those with multiple myeloma, based on the benefits demonstrated in clinical trials, and it is commonly used to realign and fix these types of spinal fractures. Radiation is occasionally combined with a kyphoplasty when the spinal cord is at risk for damage, owing to a large collection of myeloma cells within the spinal canal or involved bone pressing on the spinal cord, but most myeloma patients with vertebral fractures do not require radiation therapy to achieve both stabilization of the fracture and control of their back pain.

Other fractures or those that appear likely to break (impending fractures), such as those in the pelvis, hips, and spine, are in most cases still effectively treated with systemic therapy, although radiation therapy may also be required. Open or surgical fixation is now the exception rather than the rule in these cases.

Multiple myeloma treatment epitomizes a modern medical triumph in my opinion. This condition, which was once among the gravest of all tumors, is now very treatable, and most of the patients I care for live productive lives for many years. It is a testament to the many dedicated medical professionals that we have advanced to the current state of the art. I am quite certain that future research will yield yet more clues on how to effectively manage this condition and eventually lead to a cure.

You Have…

MULTIPLE MYELOMA!

WALDENSTROM'S MACROGLOBULINEMIA!

AMYLOIDOSIS!

MGUS!

(Monoclonal Gammopathy of Undetermined Significance)

By Robert Dolgoff, MD -- Psychiatrist

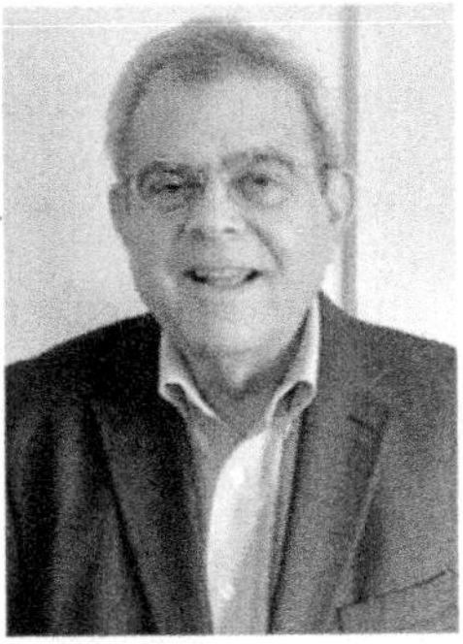

Introduction

This chapter is written from the perspective of a psychiatrist who has himself had multiple myeloma for more than six years. I was diagnosed in June 2010. I know now that I had it for some time before I was given this diagnosis. I'll say a little more about my progress with the disease later. For now, I'll let you know that despite a few crises, I have been able to maintain a good quality of life and people tell me, truthfully I think, that I look fine! Also, I've been able to continue working throughout the course of this disease with only brief periods of time when I couldn't work. As I write this chapter, I am experiencing one of a number of relapses and my treatment will soon change. So, it goes. This disease has affected me emotionally as well as physically. So far so good in both respects. Thus, I am writing as a patient and also as a psychiatrist who has over the years treated numerous people who have suffered from serious and often life-threatening diseases. Additionally, as a human being I have been part of the comings and goings of many people with severe illnesses. This chapter is infused with information gathered from all of these different life experiences.

"Beating Myeloma"

Beating myeloma? What? It's still incurable. Those of us who have multiple myeloma have to accept that while there are cures for many kinds of cancer it's likely that myeloma will be with us for the rest of our lives. This chapter is about how to deal emotionally with this frightening disease. I'll be writing to myself as well as to you. Myeloma's not a friend but it's part of me. This chapter will offer ideas about how to manage the feelings that are going to come up as we deal with this frightening disease.

We have multiple myeloma. That's cancer. "The Big C." As my friend Ira said to his family, "Bob has bone cancer!" Everyone knows what we are thinking . . . My days are numbered. I'm going to die soon. I'm going to suffer terribly. This book has accounts from many people who tell of their adventures and misadventures with myeloma. Each chapter tells another person's story and can provide guidance for you as you leave the world of the well and enter the world of the sick. My focus will mostly be on how to manage the emotional challenges that all of us face as myeloma patients. We all want to "beat cancer." Unfortunately, multiple myeloma, unlike many other cancers, remains incurable. While we can't make it go away completely, we can keep it from beating us up emotionally.

Getting The Best Possible Medical Outcome

First, of course you want to get the disease under control. What you do matters a lot. I recommend that you educate yourself about multiple myeloma so you understand what is going on in your body from the impact of this disease. You'll be getting regular updates on the results of blood tests, imaging studies, bone marrow biopsies, etc. You'll hear the names of numerous medications. It will be both confusing and at times overwhelming. The good news is that the science on MM is galloping ahead and making our lives both longer and better. It is hard to understand all the aspects that will impact your life with MM. I have a medical background but I can't understand all of it by any means. Even as a doctor, there are tests being done on my blood that I had never heard of before I was diagnosed with myeloma. The medications used to treat myeloma and prevent side effects all have at least two names—a generic name and at least one brand name. Some of those names are unpronounceable, let alone only "spellable" by your cancer expert.

New medications and combinations are appearing regularly. How can you understand the disease?

I also recommend that you see a myeloma specialist for a consultation. There are a number of them around the country. They are cancer experts who see only myeloma patients. As soon as I was told of my diagnosis by my local oncologist, he recommended that I see Dr. James Berenson in Los Angeles—that's 400 miles away from my home in Northern California. I continue to see Dr. Berenson regularly—he is on top of the newest treatments for myeloma in a way that would be impossible for any general oncologist to keep up with given the ever-increasing number of new combinations and drugs that are being tested today. Dr. Berenson gives his recommendations to my local oncologist and they discuss treatment strategies together. I have the advantage of getting treatment close to home while also getting the most up-to-date expert opinions regarding the status and treatment of my disease.

Did you know that emotional health is associated with better outcomes in cancer patients? Although not everyone believes this, there is quite a bit of evidence that it is true. People who are anxious and depressed have impairment in immune function and less resilience when faced with the stress of a serious illness.

There are a lot of resources out there; just Google multiple myeloma information or support groups and lots of useful links will appear. For starters, I can recommend Dr. James Berenson's website www.imbcr.org. This is the website for the Institute for Myeloma & Bone Cancer Research (IMBCR). Another good site is www.myelomabeacon.org. There are others as well. You won't have trouble finding information that is written in simple language that you'll be able to comprehend. Your doctor will describe different treatment options—you'll want to understand them. You'll have big decisions to make. One big decision that faces many of us early on is whether or not to have an autologous stem cell transplant. This is controversial and I won't get into that debate here. There will be other decisions as well.

I should mention here that some patients with multiple myeloma don't want to know a lot—they say, "I trust my doctor" and say, "Whatever my doctor recommends, I'll do." This was not my approach, but many people will choose this path and it is not for me to criticize this choice. This course can be tempting because in some ways it's a lot easier. I have been asked to make a lot of decisions about my choice of treatment—there are always a number of options which thankfully is growing larger every month. I could have said, "Whatever you think is best." By doing this, I would have avoided the pain of uncertainty and the worry about whether I was making the right decision. I am dealing with this anxiety right now as I face several different treatment options. Also, I am aware that by making choices myself I face the possibility that if things don't go well I might torture myself with the question "Why didn't I choose one of the other options?" Nonetheless, I'd like to feel I have some control and that my opinion counts.

What Should I Tell People?

This is a tough decision that all of us face after getting a cancer diagnosis. The disease may show on the outside or it may not. Myeloma patients may become anemic and may be pale and tired. Not infrequently myeloma patients have bone fractures and are in pain. It may not be easy to hide the fact that something is wrong but it isn't necessary to tell people the cause. Often it is quite possible to hide the fact that we have a blood cancer.

There is a definite downside to telling people. Well-meaning friends may insist you see a certain kind of healer or take an experimental remedy. They may tell you what you should and should not eat. They may say, "You don't look sick"—this is a double-edged statement. Sometimes after a cancer diagnosis "friends" will disappear from your life. This could be because they can't manage the pain or emotional upheaval they experience when thinking about cancer or interacting with a "sick person." Perhaps they themselves have lost a loved one to cancer. It could be because they are embarrassed, can't figure out what to say, and are afraid to say the wrong thing. So be it. You will have other people who will come through for you.

Then there is the question about which people to tell and which people not to tell. Certainly, almost everyone will tell close family members—parents, partners, grandparents, siblings, and children. However, this is not universally true. Did I say "close?" Once you have told selective close relatives, the rest of the relatives are likely to find out. Nonetheless, there are people who will conceal the diagnosis from certain family members, depending on the nature of the relationship with some family members and the geographical closeness or distance and the likelihood or unlikelihood that they'll find out anyway.

Beyond the circle of relatives there are close friends, neighbors, acquaintances, co-workers, and colleagues. As the circle expands, it may become more problematic to tell people and more appealing to keep your diagnosis secret. I can tell you that it can get tiresome to tell one person after another about an illness that isn't terribly rare but about which most people know just about nothing. You wind up having to reassure people that you will be okay. This is not pleasant for me as the patient!

When you're trying to live your life as a person and not a patient, you may be faced with knowing looks (or what look like knowing looks) and the inevitable question "How are you doing?" conveyed in a sympathetic way, sometimes welcome and sometimes not at all welcome. Welcome or not welcome you'll have to figure out how to respond to each such query when you might rather be living your life as a regular person rather than a "myeloma" person.

Telling people in your world about having cancer may have another potential disadvantage. People may stop trusting you to carry out your obligations and duties and they may shy away from asking you to do projects you are perfectly capable of completing. It has even happened that contracts have been taken away when a cancer diagnosis becomes known.

Once you tell a few people, you don't know how far the information will spread, so you won't know who knows and who doesn't. This can put you in an awkward position, and may interfere with friendships. Here's an example from my life. There is a work acquaintance with whom I have frequent contact and many interesting and sometimes personal conversations. I know he has cancer. Another work friend told me about it and I have no reason to believe that this is not true. Meanwhile, this person knows that I have cancer because I have been open about it with this group of people. So, he knows I have cancer, I know he has cancer, and he does not know (I think) that I know he has cancer. You might ask "So what's the problem?" Well there is no problem, but somehow it feels strange and somewhat uncomfortable to me.

Why should all of this be such a problem? I think it's because of the nature of our thinking about cancer. Until recently, many or most cancer patients had short life spans accompanied by incredible suffering and poor quality of life. If you will, cancer was considered a death sentence in more ways than one. Who wants to talk about death sentences? Now many cancers are curable and many others (like multiple myeloma) may be chronic diseases which can be managed long-term while maintaining your quality of life. In other words, as I tell many people these days, "Cancer isn't what it used to be." Despite this, public opinion has not quite caught up with this fact, and cancer is still often a word which is whispered. That's not the case with many other diseases like congestive heart failure, for example, which may be more likely to lead to incapacitating symptoms and early death.

When I was told of my diagnosis, I became frightened and I felt overwhelmed. Also, I was in a lot of pain. That was before I knew much about multiple myeloma. What to do? Of course, I told immediate family members right away. Then there was the question of what do I tell others—friends, more distant relatives, and co-workers? I decided early on that I would tell people. Of course, that was not easy—I did have to do a lot of explaining about an illness that I myself didn't understand very well. I found myself having to manage other people's feelings when I was having trouble taking care of my own. Nonetheless, the option of keeping it a secret seemed worse, especially since I knew that some people would know and others wouldn't and that could make for strange looks on some people's faces. I did tell close friends and I told people at work—both in the outpatient clinic and at the hospital where I work. The outpouring of love and support astounded me. Most, but not all, people were warm and concerned. I knew pretty quickly that I had made the right choice. Things got even better.

As my disease stabilized, people started to just go back to treating me as they always had. I haven't made a big deal out of my relapses (I have had a few); it wasn't necessary. I do get the usual questions from time to time, such as, "How are you doing?" I can tell from the tone of their voice and the look on the person's face whether it is about my myeloma or just a general question. I now mostly appreciate these questions and thank the person and say, "Fine," or, "I'm having a bit of a setback but it's manageable."

I want to mention one other outcome of my telling people about having multiple myeloma. Some people have told me they are praying for me or that a friend or family member is praying for me. Not long ago, there were reports of double-blind studies purporting to demonstrate that prayer led to better outcomes even when the patient didn't know that someone was praying for him or her. Although many people believe this, the phenomenon has not been replicated in further studies and it is no longer felt to be a scientifically proven fact. I am not a particularly religious person. Nonetheless, every time I hear about one or another person praying for me, it does make me feel good.

You might be wondering if I told my patients. I didn't. I don't think they need the burden of wondering or worrying about me, and they don't need to have feelings of uncertainty about whether I'll be there when I am needed. Of course, I could have assured them that I have great coverage in my office for this kind of thing but why even get into this? What would be the advantage? They don't come to the office to hear about me.

So, what is my conclusion about telling people? I feel happy with the choice I made but it is not the only right choice. I have tried to state the advantages and disadvantages of telling or not telling. I'm sure I haven't covered all the issues regarding this question. This is going to come down to a personal choice.

Dealing With Emotional Pain

This is certainly the hardest part. If you are made of flesh and blood, you are going to worry. You will be afraid. You will imagine the worst. You will feel alone even if you know you are deeply loved. You will brood about the future. You may question your decisions about treatment. You may have trouble sleeping and may even have sleepless nights. Steroids, which most of you will take to treat MM, are also known to interfere with sleep. You may be so preoccupied with thoughts of being ill that you lose interest in some activities that formerly were enjoyable. You may withdraw and avoid social engagements which used to be fun. All of this may occur even at times when you have no physical symptoms whatsoever. It will be more likely to occur when you are having physical discomfort or when you have just received some bad news about your lab results.

What should you do to feel better? Engage in enjoyable activities. Exercise and eat a healthy diet. Do everything your doctor tells you to do and do it faithfully. It has been demonstrated time and time again that people who take medications faithfully do better than those who miss doses or skip some medications entirely. Advocate for yourself—if you need an appointment with a medical provider because of a new symptom, you need to be persistent in asking to be seen! If your insurance gives you a hard time approving a treatment that your doctor recommends, fight it ceaselessly. This will make it more likely that you will have a good outcome medically, but will also make you feel better about yourself because you will see yourself as active and powerful. All of the above is pretty obvious. You could have written this paragraph yourself. Here are some ideas that are perhaps not so obvious:

How can you stop brooding about cancer? If there is something that is bothering you, first ask yourself whether it is a rational worry. If you think about it, you'll probably know. If it is rational, ask yourself if there is something you can do about it right now to make it better. I mean *right now.* If so, do it now. An example would be calling for an appointment with your doctor or with a specialist. If not, divert your attention to another topic.

You should also divert attention if the worry is irrational. What do I mean by diverting attention? Your mind is like a TV set. There is always a show playing—sometimes two shows with one in the background, but usually just one. We can change the channel on our TV sets, and often we can do this with our minds as well. The trick is to find a topic or activity that is exciting or compelling enough to displace the worry. Only one show should be playing and it shouldn't be the "I Have Cancer Show." Everyone has one or more ways to do this—watch an action show, sports, or a romance on TV, or a funny clip on YouTube. Read a thriller. Listen to music. Play an instrument or sing. Dance. Exercise. Meditate if that works for you. Go shopping. Play video games. Whatever! I hope you won't feel guilty about doing these things. Anything is better than letting your mind loop endlessly and pointlessly about being sick. I'm doing this right now as I write this chapter—remember when I told you I am in a challenging situation right now with my own myeloma? It may sound corny, but it works. I go through this exercise with patients in my office with some regularity. Sometimes they claim there is nothing that can divert their attention. When we look carefully, we always find something that will work for at least a short period of time. Pick something that's easy to do. Pick a passive activity that doesn't take much effort – it's easier to turn on the TV than to start a new book, and easier to listen to music than to exercise. Yes, the worry will come back, but then the channel can be changed again for a while. I'm not promising magical permanent relief from worry.

A few other tips—be nice to yourself! Buy the pleasurable item that you thought you shouldn't. Yes, you ought to save money for treatment or for your heirs, but do you really think you need to do that? Even a small present for yourself will feel really good. If you saved money throughout your life, why did you do it? Isn't it there for a time like this? If you need to take pain medication, take it—don't just tough it out and continue to feel poorly.

Emotional support from other people is also very helpful. For years, I regularly read and posted on the ACOR myeloma blog, but that blog shut down. Now I subscribe to the Myeloma Beacon (myelomabeacon.org). People with myeloma tell their stories, report on treatments and side effects, and write about their personal joys and struggles. It's educational and reassuring, although it can also be sad and upsetting. Be careful, as sometimes the information can be misleading. If you are not sure, ask your doctor. Regardless, you won't feel alone, and that's very important. You will also probably be able to find an in-person multiple myeloma support group in your area. Many of them meet once a month and invite speakers, and participants trade stories and support.

You may want to see a psychotherapist. There are many kinds of psychotherapists. I recommend seeing someone who encourages you to talk about what is going on in the here and now. One who can help you devise practical strategies regarding how to deal with emotional pain or with your relationships with others that may have been difficult for a long time, or are just now becoming difficult as you deal with your illness.

While it's normal to feel discouraged, sad, and worried, be alert to the possibility that you may have fallen into a real clinical depression. You can identify this by looking for the following symptoms—self-criticism, feelings of hopelessness, loss of interest in all or nearly all activities, and pervasive sadness or worry that is always there and won't go away. A clinical depression can be treated successfully with medications that may be prescribed by a psychiatrist or by your primary care physician or nurse practitioner. Some oncologists may be comfortable prescribing some psychiatric medications. Of course, just as with cancer, there's a stigma about depressive and anxiety disorders and taking medications for them—people don't want to talk about these conditions and they feel that nothing will help. Not true for cancer, and not true for these emotional disturbances.

To summarize, just because a disease is incurable doesn't mean that you can't beat it. Certainly, emotionally, you can keep it from beating you. Even if it winds up shortening your life, it need not ruin it. Get as much information about the disease as you can and be an active participant in planning treatment. See a myeloma specialist, even if it means traveling to another city for the consultation. Remind yourself always that cancer is not what it used to be. This is especially true of multiple myeloma which today is usually a chronic disease which can be managed successfully. If you have had myeloma for a few years, you have probably already experienced its downs and ups. If you have reason to think that your emotional pain is unmanageable, then seek help from a mental health professional who has had experience dealing with people with medical illnesses. You'll want to think about your illness, and you'll want to understand it as well as possible, but you should not think about it too much. Most of all, remember that you are much more than a patient—you are a person with a life to live quite apart from the demands of this uninvited guest called multiple myeloma. Maybe you can't actually beat myeloma in the sense of making it go away, but you can keep it from beating you.

You Have…

MULTIPLE MYELOMA!

WALDENSTROM'S MACROGLOBULINEMIA!

AMYLOIDOSIS!

MGUS!

(Monoclonal Gammopathy of Undetermined Significance)

By Xiuling Ma, PhD, OMD -- Acupuncturist

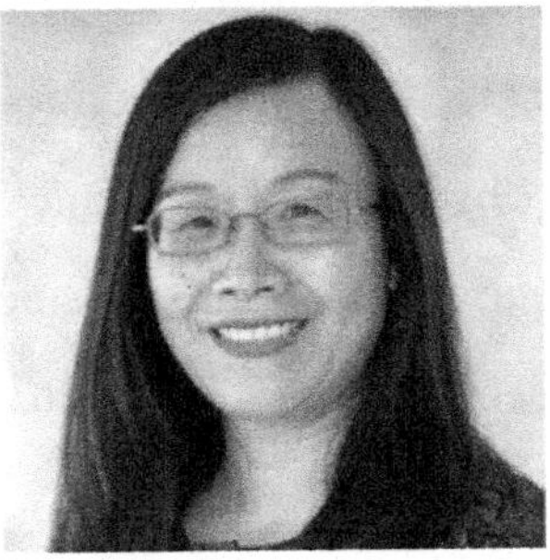

Acupuncture can help regulate the immune system by promoting the movement of lymph glands and blood. It is helpful in treating the specific symptoms that arise from MM, MGUS, Waldenstrom's macroglobulinemia, and amyloidosis; and, therefore, is very helpful as an adjunctive therapy. Patients undergoing chemotherapy or surgery heal faster and feel better with acupuncture.

Acupuncture helps to reduce the side effects of these treatments without reducing their efficacy, and is one of the best modalities for the treatment of pain and neuropathy. It is highly recommended to try acupuncture as replacement for pain medications, because it can help the body heal as it takes away the pain sensation. Also, many patients deal with anxiety and insomnia due to the challenges that they and their family must face with these diseases. Acupuncture can help with these issues, significantly improving the quality of life of patients and strengthening their mental and physical states.

Along with acupuncture, herbal medicine offers many benefits. The combination of herbal medicine with acupuncture is a time-tested medicine which provides so much relief and healing for patients. And like acupuncture, herbs can also be extremely helpful for patients dealing with the side effects of chemotherapy, surgery, and radiation, and certain herbs can also help with blood production. While some people are concerned about the quality of the herbs, there are actually many herbal companies which exceed the highest standards for herbal supplements. Chinese herbal medicine has been refined through thousands and thousands of years of observation and clinical practice. Our herbs are very safe and effective, with time-tested herbal combinations that can be tailored to each patient's individual symptoms and constitution.

Although some doctors have concerns about the interactions of Western medicine and traditional herbs, I have seen how well they can work together. There is a lot of information available. We know which herbs shouldn't be combined with certain Western medications. Though they are both extremely important, there are even times when herbal remedies are actually the better choice. For more chronic issues, herbs can be the better option because you can take them for longer periods of time without causing side effects.

According to Chinese medicine, health is defined as a balanced physical, mental, and energetic state, and from the TCM (Traditional Chinese Medicine) perspective, disease is caused by physical and energetic imbalances within the body. Acupuncture is one of the few tools able to treat these physical and energetic aspects of disease, and promote emotional and psychological well-being. This is of paramount importance for patients.

I approach each patient as an individual. I look at the patient's health as a whole. I want to know how their digestion is doing, and if they have a good appetite. I want to know how they are sleeping. I want to know about their emotional well-being, along with their physical symptoms. I will also use objective tests such as pulse analysis and tongue diagnosis to help make a treatment plan. I will factor in all of this when I make a diagnosis. My treatments focus on relieving specific complaints while also promoting the patient's overall health. Ultimately, my goal is to enhance the conventional treatment and reduce any side effects the patient might be dealing with.

Most of the time, I see patients at my office, and therefore don't get a chance to see family and caregivers. However, if the patient wants them to come along, it can be very helpful to hear from people who live or work closely with the patient.

Regarding treatment options, I provide acupuncture, herbal medicine, and dietary recommendation. I also use cupping, manual therapy, meditation or moving meditation, and infrared therapy if it's appropriate for the patient.

To reduce the risks of developing problems and to improve the patient's outcome, it is important to relieve stress and have good eating habits. Moderate exercise, meditation, relaxation practices, and a good sleep schedule are also helpful. Hard work and vigorous exercise should be postponed until after recovery. Spending time with loved ones and enjoying life will help the body heal. The exact food to eat depends on each person but eating unprocessed and organic foods is the best choice. Also, eating more cooked meals is better than raw meals. This helps aid digestion.

I recommend that sugary foods should be avoided as much as possible. Overly rich and greasy foods, such as fried foods and cheese, should also be cut out of the diet. Patients should immediately stop any illegal substances as well as alcohol and tobacco. If there is constipation, eating asparagus and other high-fiber vegetables will help promote a bowel movement. Jujube can help promote new blood cell growth for patients dealing with anemia. There are many herbs that can help with the treatment process, but it depends on the individual. I would recommend seeing a licensed practitioner trained in herbal medicine.

There are other practices that can help patients. Qi Gong is a very healthy practice. It is similar to Tai Chi, but with more of a focus on promoting health. Qi Gong is an ancient medical exercise technique designed to promote circulation and calm the mind. I teach specific Qi Gong movements to my patients to help them overcome their illness.

My advice to patients would be to stay positive and upbeat. Try your best to laugh and enjoy yourself, because this will help you overcome whatever challenge you are facing. As hard as it is, it is very important to put very demanding projects on hold until after you are feeling better. Do the things you enjoy while also making sure to not overstrain or tax your body. Eat well, get good rest, meditate, and remain in a relaxed state of mind as much as possible. Being in nature is a very healing thing to do that people often forget about. Taking the time to walk in the park or take a light hike can be very beneficial. The body is very resilient and there are many things we can do to help the recovery process.

Working with other healthcare professionals is very important. Acupuncture and herbal medicine should always be combined with Western treatment protocols for these illnesses. I try to keep a dialogue with my fellow practitioners so they know what I'm doing and what my assessment of the patient is. I greatly appreciate feedback and data from the patient's other healthcare providers. Medicine works better when multiple treatment modalities are combined together. What one modality lacks, another will be help, and vice versa. I recommend that patients seek out assistance from multiple sources, as long as they are well-established medical disciplines.

EPILOGUE

I hope that you have found this book useful in learning more about multiple myeloma, Waldenstrom's macroglobulinemia, amyloidosis, and MGUS from the patient, caregiver, and healthcare professional perspectives. This book is not a substitute for getting your own medical advice. Always consult your doctor to get the care that is right for you. The information provided here should help you, your family, and your caregivers achieve the best life possible while coping with one of these diseases. This book offers not only information, but also provides reassurance that your life with these disorders can be fulfilling and long-lasting. I also wish to convey that the future is bright, as more effective therapies are becoming available nearly every month for treating these diseases, which certainly will continue the dramatic improvement in the lives of patients.

ABOUT THE AUTHOR

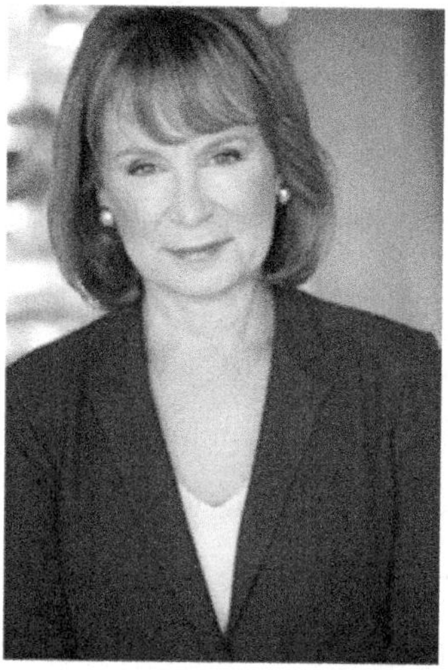

Debra is a professional actress and a member of both SAG-AFTRA and Actors Equity. She has been seen and heard in numerous TV, movie, and stage productions, TV and radio commercials, and voice-overs. She received her BFA cum laude from the University of Southern California and has Certificates of Completion from Cambridge University in Cambridge, England and the Royal Academy of Dramatic Arts in London, England. She is president and founder of Performing Artists Against Cancer. Debra is a proud third-generation life member of Hadassah; to carry on the tradition, she made both of her daughters fourth-generation members of Hadassah.

Debra is also a classical pianist and performed a benefit recital for the Institute for Myeloma & Bone Cancer Research (IMBCR) on the great Vladimir Horowitz' piano during "The Legendary Steinway Pianos Tour." She serves as a patient advocate for Berenson Oncology and is also the Event Chair for the IMBCR's Advisory Committee, overseeing event planning and helping produce its many benefits, including comedy at the Skirball Cultural Center with Renée

Taylor & Joseph Bologna; jazz at The Catalina Bar & Grill with Bennie Maupin & Todd Cochran, and another benefit there starring "The All-Star Jazz Ensemble" with Lance Crane; a benefit performed by five-time Grammy award nominee and 38-time Gold- and Platinum-certified guitarist Ottmar Liebert at the Hopmonk Tavern in Sebastopol, CA; art at the Andrew Weiss Gallery (Marilyn Monroe photos and Picasso pottery); and film benefits, one as part of the Los Angeles Indian Film Festival in Cooking with Stella starring Lisa Ray, and another with the premiere of Love is All You Need starring Pierce Brosnan.

She has been married to Dr. James Berenson for more than 39 years. They have two daughters, Ariana Berenson and Shira Berenson Feinstein, a son-in-law, Dr. Aaron Feinstein, and a newly adopted dog, (Teddy) Bear.

28421252R00241

Made in the USA
Columbia, SC
10 October 2018